Published by GLS Publications, Clayhall, Essex

First Printed in Great Britain in September 2000
Second Edition Printed in May 2002

This book has been printed on environmentally-friendly paper

ABOUT THE AUTHOR

Dr Gina Shaw, M.A., AIYS (Dip. Irid.) was awarded a BA (Hons) in Applied Philosophy with Criminology in 1997, a Master of Arts award with Merit in Applied Philosophy in 1999, and a Doctor of Science award in the year 2000 as a Doctor of Complementary Medicine. She is also a qualified Iridologist. Dr Shaw is a lecturer of health and nutritional science and provides certification courses in Life Science, lectures around the country and personal health and nutritional consultations by telephone, email and in person. She also provides fasting supervision and iridology consultations and now has a health retreat in Devon.

Dr Shaw has published other books including 'The Dangers of Pharmaceutical and Herbal Drugs and the Fallacy of Animal Experimentation', a philosophical book entitled 'Animal Intelligence: An Amazing Insight into the Abilities of Animals and its Implications' 'The Healthy Vegan Child' and 'Quick and Easy Raw Recipes for Maximum Nutrition'.

If you would like more information about regaining your health, courses in Natural Health, health retreats or information about other books and articles by the author, please contact
True Health, c/o 8 Marston Road, Clayhall, Essex IG5 OLZ
or telephone (01626) 352765
DrGinaShaw@aol.com/www.vibrancy.homestead.com/pageone.html

A SPECIAL DEDICATION

I would like to dedicate this book to my dearest darling Jet, whom I will never forget and will always love. You gave me so much in your life and for this I will always be grateful. Your sweet nature is something I will remember so fondly and you will always be missed.

ACKNOWLEDGEMENTS

I would also like to thank those people around me who care for me and support me in my work, including my mother, Mrs Anita Shaw, and my father, Mr Harry Shaw, and my partner Matthew Cooper. Mum and Dad your love for me is greatly valued, beyond words. I only hope you have the strength of character necessary to turn around your lives in the way myself, my clients and so many others have too.

Matthew, the wisdom you have often astounds me and I hope we can continue learning together and supporting one another despite the struggles which sometimes surround us.

PREFACE

A need for the collective human consciousness to elevate itself from the complacency of familiar social behaviours, and rise to the calling of a heightened global, as well as personal responsibility, has reached a crisis point. Time is no longer a human asset, but a concept of cognitive perception that is rapidly becoming an endangered dimension.

There is an endless stream of books pandering to the weaknesses of those too complacent to receive anything other than a 'pat on the back' for their inconsequential efforts in adopting more healthful personal habits. Each of these volumes fuels the fire of the collective apathy that is currently poisoning and destroying all life on earth. We can no longer afford to rely on the fringe-dwelling minority of the population to courageously pursue their inquiring minds, and divert us all from the path of personal and global destruction. The time has come for collaboration between all those who have the ability of using their knowledge and courage to bring sense to the senseless. The potential of humans to experience superb health will never be realized until the tried and failed formula of money and technological hierarchy has been replaced with one of education coupled with authentic personal responsibility toward all life.

The monstrous dams built in order to divert, and thus control, the blood flow of our mother earth represent a living analogy for the way in which the path of money, in itself an innocent token of value, has been perverted into a force capable of destroying all that it was designed to represent. The roots of financial exchange were long ago ripped from the soil of its innocent intent and plunged into a sewer of obsessional control and greed. The wake of money is one of fragmented and denatured morals, abuse, pain and suffering. Nowhere is this more evidently manifest than in the adhesiveness of the medical approach to health, and the sticky sickness of mass dietary habits.

Individual disempowerment and apathy, born of cultural dogma, have accelerated and accumulated over the centuries. They have led us down a path towards pending personal, collective and global disaster.

Spirituality and science dine together at the table of salvation, and we are invited to join them providing we adopt the appropriate attire. Courage to think independently of collective perceptions, strength to stand independently of system driven lifestyle choices, and a commitment to living parallel to our knowledge, are all necessary qualities if health and survival are to be our prizes. Knowledge is the golden key to transformation, turned by the hand of need. A shift in personal consciousness is ignited when a window of opportunity arises. Such a window, along with the knowledge to inspire change, can be found on every page of this book. Dr Gina Shaw deserves applause for putting into print the truths that few want to learn of, let alone acknowledge, accept, embrace or, above all, respond to.

It is a myth that the terrible sufferings of animals farmed for human consumption are contained within the walls of the slaughterhouse. Their pain can be found echoing and resonating in the chests of cardiac patients; their cries for help heard as another bone breaks in those with osteoporosis; their terror can be seen in the faces of those diagnosed with cancer, and their hopelessness felt in the flaccid limbs of stroke patients.

I encourage you, the reader, to rise to the unwritten challenge posed by the author of this potentially life-changing book. The challenge is to transcend mass apathy and commonly accepted modes and codes of immoral and destructive dietary choices. I encourage you to reclaim your health, while simultaneously reducing the suffering of all life. I support you and wholeheartedly encourage you to step beyond your own system-indoctrinated comfort zone so that you may reach for that which your body yearns, your mind understands, and your soul knows is right.

Professor Rozalind A. Gruben A.H.S.I., R.S.A.

CONTENTS

SECTION ONE

SCIENTIFIC REASONS FOR AVOIDING MEAT

INTRODUCTION

Did you know that the two leading causes of death in the U.S. are directly related to the consumption of meat? When I use the term meat, in order to clear up any confusion anyone may have, I am referring to all animal flesh, be it from cows, turkeys, pigs, chickens, fish, in fact, any animal that lives and breaths and that humans consume! I am talking about all animal flesh.

Although the arguments in this book are concerned with a meat-free diet, you will realise from this book that a diet *free of all animal products* is highly recommended for health reasons, as well as for ethical, religious and environmental reasons. Indeed, cutting out meat and animal products such as dairy, eggs, honey, gelatine, and other slaughterhouse scraps greatly reduces the likelihood of generating debilitating and deadly diseases.

Upon reading this book, you will find study after study, performed over the years on often very large populations which prove time and time again that a meat-based diet is not only dangerous, but that it also has the potential to decrease one's lifespan and quality of life dramatically. Although, a meat-based diet has never been suited to humans due to their anatomical and physiological make-up, it must be conceded that, in more recent years, it has taken an even greater toll on the meat-eating populations of the World. Nowadays, practically all animals are intensively-reared; they are cramped in squalid conditions and are subject to unnatural and extremely abusive conditions, including so-called free range animals (see Penman, 1996 for further details). To top this, they are fed largely unnatural diets often comprising of other diseased animals, as well as many chemical concoctions.

Patrice Green, J.D., M.D. and Allison Lee Solin state([1]) that animal products easily account for our largest intake of pesticides and herbicides, in fact, more than 80 to 90 percent by some estimates. Factory-farmed animals (raised in over-crowded confinement systems) are fed cheap feed containing pesticide-ridden grains, antibiotics, and often the remains of other animals. Each time an animal ingests pesticides, the residues of those chemicals build up in the animal's body tissues since they are bombarded with these chemicals day after day. This process is called 'bioaccumulation' and occurs especially with persistent chemicals such as organochlorines (a group that includes DDT).

In her book 'Hormone Deception'([7]), D. Lindsey Berkson states that eating high in the food chain runs you into all sorts of problems. Meat and dairy consistently have the highest levels of persistent hormone disruptors for a number of reasons, including:

1. Oestrogenic hormones or growth enhancers given to cattle, pigs and poultry in order that they grow bigger and fatter faster. These growth hormones are also given to dairy cows to up their production of milk.
2. Conventional animal feeds are among the most heavily sprayed crops. Most animal feed is laced with pesticides, herbicides and fungicides, many of which are being investigated as hormone disruptors. Toxins, such as pesticides and drug residues, concentrate in animal fat. According to the EPA, 90-95% of all pesticide residues are found in meat and dairy products.
3. Most animal feed contains rendered fat (fat salvaged from fast-food restaurants and animal houses, often laced with melted plastic, etc.) and is a source of disrupting chemicals dissolved into the fat. This can wreak havoc with the consumer's hormones.

Also, growth promoting hormones are placed as pellets in the ear's of cattle and are supposed to be removed five days before slaughter, in countries such as the U.S. It's possible that not all the hormone residues have left the cattle's body after only five days. Animals, like humans, don't all metabolise hormones at exactly the same time. Also, the pellets may not always be removed. Since oestrogenic hormones store in fat and meat is a high-fat food, just removing the pellets doesn't mean all the residues stored in the animal's fat will be gone.

Meat also has antibiotic residues. One half of all antibiotics in the U.S.

alone are used in the production of livestock. Antibiotics too can contribute to hormone-disruptor exposure.

In 1998, the U.S. Food and Drug Administration (FDA) detected dangerous pesticides such as malathion and chlorpyrifos-methyl in animal feed. Pesticides in animal feed are only just the beginning though, as the reader will learn. The intensive way factory-farmed animals are raised means that plagues can travel quickly through a farm, leading to a heavy reliance on pesticides, antibiotics, and other drugs. For example, factory farmers most commonly use pesticides and larvicides to control fly populations drawn by so many animals and so much manure.

As biologist Sandra Steingraber noted in her 1997 book 'Living Downstream', the largest contributors to daily intake of chlorinated insecticides are dairy products, meat, fish and poultry.

A recent article from ABC News entitled 'High Dioxin Levels Found in Food' reports that Americans are getting 22 times the maximum dioxin exposure suggested by the U.S. Environmental Protection Agency[2]. The scientists say that levels of dioxin, among the most toxic substances on earth, remain high in the U.S. food supply although they have declined in the environment. Similar situations will naturally arise in the food supply of other civilised nations. Dioxins, contained in Agent Orange, are a toxic chemical known for causing various forms of cancer. Occasional natural occurences, such as volcanic eruptions or forest fires, can also produce them.

Indeed, in food samples from around the U.S., scientists at the University of Texas School of Public Health at Houston found no decline from test samples taken more than a decade ago. "It means we still have to tighten up and clean up our environment more than it is right now" said Dr. Arnold Schecter, who directed the study. "We have to reduce the highly toxic, persistent chemicals in the environment.". Conversely, blood samples from pure vegans who consume no animal products, show that they have less dioxins in their bodies than average Americans.

As if that isn't enough, in a recent article entitled 'Meat Your Death?'[4] by Lawrence J. Jacobs, M.D., and Caroline Kweller, they report that a survey by Public Citizen, the Government Accountability Project, and the American

5

Federation of Government Employees, found that 46 percent of federal inspectors had been unable to recall meat laden with animal faeces, vomit, metal shards, and other contamination. In 1998 USDA (United States Department of Agriculture) declared safe for human consumption animal carcasses carrying a host of diseases, such as cancers, tumours, open sores, poultry pneumonia, infection arthritis, and diseases caused by intestinal worms. Workers can simply cut off visibly affected areas, and the meat counts as approved. Furthermore, from the year 2001 the USDA imposed rules that classify as 'safe for human consumption' slaughterhouse products with certain illnesses and sores including cancer, intestinal worms, sores, infectious arthritis, glandular swellings and airsacculitis (pneumonia of poultry). Apparently, these diseases do not prevent a health risk(!)[5]).

In fact, Delmar Jones, a veteran federal food inspector from Renlap, Alabama, is so revolted by filth he sees on the job that he has refused to eat meat, he said in a mid-2000 news interview. He is trying to get his wife to stop, too: "I've told her what she's eating." "Veterinarians are now approving cattle that wheeze loudly as they're breathing before slaughter and whose lungs are filled with fluid; they have scar tissue and abscesses running all up and down the sides of their lungs....Other cattle are approved that are stuffed with regurgitated food that was oozing out. Faecal smears up to a foot long, along with hair, grubs, adhesions, fluke, and ingesta, are all getting on the line," read some excerpts from the letter.

Foodborne diseases such as campylobacter, listeria, E. coli, and salmonella affect millions of Americans and Britons each year and kill more than 5,000, particularly children, the elderly, and those with weak immune systems. In the vast majority of cases, people contract these diseases after eating animal products—meat, poultry, eggs, and dairy—or from items contaminated by animal products or animal faeces.

Whatever nutrients may be found in animal food, it is not worth the stress put on the body and the energy required to extract them. Animal food is highly acid-forming and, according to Dr Robert Young, a microbiologist and nutritionist from the U.S., has high levels of bacteria, yeast/fungus and associated toxins. The methods involved in using domesticated animals for human food involve a number of steps which increase exposure to yeast/fungus and their mycotoxins. Some animals eat stored feed such as silos which is characteristically fungally contaminated and toxic. These influences are passed to the consumer according to Dr Young([6]).

Cooked animal foods are dead, enzymatically-speaking. They lack enzymes which help us to break down foodstuff, the lack phytonutrients which are by their very nature abundant in fresh, raw plant foods and they lack many essential vitamins and minerals.

Some people might be thinking to themselves, 'Well, maybe if I ate free-range meat or organic meat, I would be better off'. Well, after years of studying the subject of flesh foods and its causal relationship with health, the evidence, based on our anatomy and physiology, suggests that even eating these type of 'alternative meats' would definitely not add up to a healthy diet, no matter how healthy the animals were, and no matter what idyllic conditions that the animals were kept in. In fact, the implications would not be much better at all. In a recent report by Dr Green and Solin they argue that organic meat, dairy and eggs certainly cannot be held to be a healthy option as not only do animal products contain cholesterol, and are typically high in fat, they have been found to significantly raise risks for heart disease, stroke, hypertension, obesity and cancer([1]).

From this book, the reader shall see that the digestive apparatus of humans is definitely not suited to a meat-based diet, and meat will inevitably poison the human organism. The fact is that whether people eat organic or commercially-produced meat, most people who consume flesh foods and its products are in a state of pregnant ill health; disease is just waiting to manifest. The symptoms may not be there, but the toxic state is ever present.

Free-range farms are supposed to mean that the animals are allowed to roam freely, but in some commercial farms it means an open pen of 50,000 birds in the same building with access to barren fenced yards. Too many birds in one open space will fight, so they are debeaked (without anaesthetic), which is common practice in non-organic and non-free-range commercial poultry farms. Without beaks the birds cannot eat whole grain and are fed only pellets of refined foods laced with rendered fat. Since birds (chickens and turkeys) are fed this type of cheap feed are rather tasteless, more fat (such as coconut oil) is injected into their flesh during processing, thus poultry can end up being much higher in fat than is commonly assumed[7].

It is interesting to note that as far back as 1991 the World Health Organisation called for an end to the promotion of meat and dairy products and insisted on a revolution in agricultural policies away from livestock and towards plants. This advice, however, was largely ignored. And in 1995, the Oxford Study gave us even more to think about when they announced that there were 20 percent lower premature deaths amongst vegetarians - in other words, **vegetarians live longer than meat-eaters[3]**. Unfortunately, some of the many studies are never noticed by the public for various political and financial reasons. However, the author feels that it is high time that the results of these studies were noticed, taken in and acted upon for the sake of the human race and the planet!

I sincerely hope that, upon reading this book, you will not only benefit yourself in your quest towards superior health and well-being, but also you will pass on to others the valuable information contained in this book. If you are currently a meat-eater and are hoping to change your eating patterns, this book should provide you with a new impetus for change. If, however, you are already consuming a healthy diet - one which is free of all animal products, I hope you might see that increasing your intake of raw food would improve your health dramatically.

CHAPTER ONE: SCIENTIFIC REASONS FOR AVOIDING MEAT

In this chapter, we will be concerned with the anatomical, physiological, pathological and nutritional reasons for eliminating flesh foods from our diet, and why optimal health is not possible on a meat-based diet. The discussion will focus on the health problems that can be caused by the consumption of flesh foods, and the vibrant health that can be attained (or regained) by adherence to a plant-based diet, particularly that which is not only devoid of flesh foods or flesh products, but also one which is based predominantly on raw, ripe fruits and vegetables and nuts and seeds.

The Best Fuel for the Human Body
From about 24 to 5 million years ago, fruits appear to have been the main dietary constituent for hominids, according to Boyd and Konner[8]. Indeed, this was confirmed back in May 1977 when The New York Times featured an article about some findings by Dr Alan Walker of the John Hopkins University in Maryland who had discovered paleontological evidence of our early human diet. He discovered, from fossilised evidence that early man had been a fruit-eater, in fact, not only a fruit-eater, but exclusively a fruit-eater. Early man ate nothing but fruit! By the careful examination of fossilised teeth and human remains, and with the aid of electron microscopy and other sophisticated apparatus, Dr Walker and his colleagues concluded that they had definite evidence of the fact that earliest human life ate only fruit. From a Darwinian perspective, this would be quite a natural assumption, given our extremely close genetic links with other primates (we share 98.4% of our genetic DNA with chimpanzees), and in particular bonobos (pygmy chimps) who survive on large quantities of fruit and raw plants and, incidentally, who have never been known to hunt. Indeed, we are the only species who cook our food and, as a consequence of this, we are seeing an increasing amount of degenerative diseases under a myriad of names, with new ones created regularly[1].

The human body can be maintained on a conglomerate assortment of foods, otherwise our race would have long since vanished; but it does so to our own detriment. A car can run on kerosene, but it will clog up, parts will wear out sooner and its serviceable life will be greatly reduced. Likewise, the human body will also work best and last longest on the fuel intended for humans: raw fruits, raw vegetables and raw unsalted nuts and seeds. The biology of humans is such that the body is much more capable of obtaining complete and optimal nutrition, without threat or stress, from plant foods[1].

All nutritive material is formed in the plant kingdom and animals have the capacity to appropriate, but never to form or create food elements. Plants can synthesise amino acids from air, earth and water, but all animals (including humans) are dependent upon plant protein, either directly by eating the plant, or indirectly by eating an animal which has eaten the plant. Out of the amino acids found in plant and/or animal tissues used as food, the living organism synthesises the numerous proteins needed by the cells and tissues of its own body. There are no amino acids in flesh that the animal did not derive from the plant and that man cannot also derive from the plant.

The problem is, of course, that those who eat animals get only the nutritional elements which the animals have obtained from vegetation, which have deteriorated with the impurities and putrescence invariably present in man's blood and tissues, as a result of consuming animal flesh. When you eat foods from the plant kingdom, you receive amino acids in ideal combinations with other substances which are essential to the full utilisation of protein, carbohydrates, minerals, vitamins, enzymes, hormones - in addition to chlorophyl, which only plants can supply. The best sources of concentrated protein for man are raw, unsalted nuts and seeds - the amino acids are wholesomely alive and unchanged. **Raw plant foods contain all the vitamins, minerals, trace elements, carbohydrates, hormones and enzymes necessary for the human organism to produce tissue and other body constituents of the highest quality.**

However, it has been amply shown that the habitual consumption of meat (which includes red meat, white meat, poultry and fish) is actually one of the main causes of degenerative disease. The total elimination of flesh foods from the diet is one of the most important steps towards gaining (or regaining) optimal health. The reason behind this is simple: Our anatomy and physiology are poorly adapted to the processing of meat and, therefore, flesh foods cannot be digested without some putrefaction (in addition to the putrefaction already present in the meat itself). This inevitably leads to toxaemia, which is the starting point of degenerative diseases like gout, arthritis, heart disease, hardening of the arteries, and stroke, osteoporosis, cancer, etc.

Our Anatomy & Physiology

Our anatomy and digestive system are totally dissimilar to those of carnivores. Carnivores have sharp claws and teeth for killing and tearing, they have short intestinal canals and strong secretions of hydrochloric acid, so as to quickly digest and expel the waste products of the flesh they consume, before putrefaction can occur. Carnivores are able to secrete an enzyme called uricase which breaks down uric acid, from flesh foods, into a harmless substance called allantoin, however, humans do not possess this enzyme. If we partake in our natural diet of raw vegetable proteins, for instance by consuming nuts and seeds, these foodstuffs contain enough carbohydrates to render this enzyme unnecessary[1].

To demonstrate the unsuitability of humans bodies' to flesh foods, let us look a little deeper into our physiology. The length of the alimentary canal is approximately three times the length of the body in carnivorous animals, ten times the length of the body in the omnivore and twelve times the length of the body in the anthropoid apes, which includes us, humans. These figures are approximate and, in fact, some books give the length of the human alimentary canal as approximately thirty feet, but the fact of the matter is that the alimentary canal of human beings is comparable only to anthropoid apes who are frugivores by nature (Ibid.). Therefore, rapidly putrefying flesh foods have the ability to cause havoc in our digestive system.

There are also other facts which make flesh foods a very poor option for the human body. The human digestive tract is sacculated, for the express purpose of retaining the food as long as possible in the intestine until all possible nutriment has been extracted from it, and our gastric juices contain less germicidal and antiseptic properties than a carnivore's. These are the worst possible conditions for the processing of flesh foods. **Thus, rapidly decaying flesh foods will most likely putrefy in the human digestive tract (Ibid.).**

Another concern would be regarding the excessive secretion of bile (necessitated for the digestion of flesh foods) which may result in the premature breakdown of the liver and the large quantities of uric acid created by a flesh diet may have disastrous effects on the kidneys. Dr Robert Perk says that the excess of uric acid "causes contraction of the minute blood vessels, resulting in high arterial tension and often the blocking of the blood vessels by the uric acid. This results in serious interference with the circulation and blood supply to the tissues and throws great strain on the vital organs, especially the heart and kidneys." (cited in [1]).

Meat is the most putrefactive of all foods. **This means that meat is more liable to decay in the human gastro-intestinal tract than any other food.** Flesh, when it is eaten by humans, tends to undergo a process of decay in the stomach or intestinal tract causing a poisoning of the blood. Putrefaction in meat-eaters is evidenced by bad breath, heartburn, eructations and smelly stools and it is probable that the attempts of the body to eliminate these wastes has a profound influence on the shortening of our life span (Ibid.).

If the body fluid that bathes our cells is overloaded with waste, causing an excessive secretion of bile, fatigue, weakening and ageing are the inevitable results. The accumulation of toxic substances in the body causes the deterioration of the intestinal flora and the blood vessels gradually lose their natural elasticity - their walls become hardened and thickened. Irreversible damage to the organism will then inevitably occur (Ibid.).

Health Problems
The hardest thing for the human body to digest is cooked animal protein - it leaves us feeling very weak and tired. Protein, being the most complex of all food elements, makes its utilization the most

12

complicated. Those people with an impaired digestion will find it preferable to ingest a lesser quantity of concentrated protein of which they will be more capable of utilizing, rather than a greater quantity which not only cannot be processed efficiently, but which may poison the body.

When protein is eaten in greater amounts than the body is capable of utilising, the organism is subjected to the toxic by-products of protein metabolism, which it has been unable to eliminate - and the inevitable result is degenerative disease[1].

As mentioned, meat passes very slowly through the human digestive system which is not designed to digest it. In fact, flesh foods can take about 5 days to pass out of the body (plant foods take about 1½ days). During this time the disease-causing products of decaying meat are in constant contact with the digestive organs. The habit of eating animal flesh in its characteristic state of decomposition creates a poisonous state in the colon and wears out the intestinal tract prematurely (Ibid.).

Often poisonous bacteria present in flesh foods are not destroyed by cooking, especially if the meat is undercooked, barbecued, or roasted on a spit - these are notorious sources of infection. The stomach will attempt to break down animal flesh with chemicals which are ill-equipped to handle flesh foods as we have such a low amount of hydrochloric acid, as compared with carnivorous animals. This hydrochloric acid we do have is also low in acidity, as compared to a carnivorous animal. Next, the animal flesh passes into the small intestine until it comes to the ileocaecal valve. Passing through the ileocecal valve it enters the caecum which is at the base of the ascending colon. From here the second stage of digestion starts. The chime becomes a seething mass of intestinal flora. When dead bodies are incorporated in our food, the flora is putrefactive and their mission is to destroy. From the colon, they are drawn into the bloodstream by suction and, as they circulate around the body, disease or sickness is the inevitable result (Ibid.). On a fruit and vegetation diet, the natural flora are fermentative and break down this type of food - they are not pathogenic and are quite harmless to the body for the simply reason that we are not flesh eaters([2]).

British and American Scientists who have studied intestinal bacteria of meat-eaters as compared to vegetarians have found significant differences. The bacteria in the meat eaters' intestines react with digestive juices to produce chemicals which have been found to cause bowel cancer. This may explain why cancer of the bowel is very prevalent in meat-eating areas like North America and Western Europe, while it is extremely rare in vegetarian countries such as India. In the US, bowel cancer is the second most common form of cancer (second only to lung cancer). Conversely, recent studies have found that chicken meat is the most carcinogenic meat that people can eat due to the amount of the carcinogen (toxic compound) PhIP contained in it - although, as we will find, all meat is dangerous and carcinogenic to the human body. (More information about the links between chicken meat and cancer can be found later on).

Another important point is that meat contains waste products that the animal did not get to eliminate, and toxic hormones and fluids released into the bloodstream and tissues at the moment of the death of the terrified animal. This is commonly referred to as 'pain poisoning'. An animal's cellular life continues after death. The cells continue to produce waste materials which are trapped in the blood and decaying tissues. The nitrogenous extracts which are trapped in the animal's muscles are partially responsible for the flavour of the cooked meat. Just before and during the agony of being slaughtered, the biochemistry of the terrified animal undergoes profound changes. During times of intense rage or fear, animals, no less than humans, undergo profound biochemical changes in dangerous situations. The hormone level in the animal's blood - especially the hormone adrenaline - changes radically as they see other animals dying around them and they struggle futilely for life and freedom. These large amounts of hormones remain in the meat and later poison the human tissue. According to the Nutrition Institute of America "The flesh of an animal carcass is loaded with toxic blood and other waste by-products"(cited in [1]).

14

Therefore, the fact is that toxic by-products are forced throughout the body, thus poisoning the entire carcass. The flesh is invaded by a putrefactive virus which are nature's scavengers to get rid of dead bodies. As soon as an animal is killed, proteins in its body coagulate, and self-destruct enzymes are released (unlike slow decaying plants which have a rigid cell wall). Soon denatured substances called ptomaines are formed. Due to these ptomaines that are released immediately after death, animal flesh and eggs have a common property - extremely rapid decomposition and putrefaction. By the time the animal is slaughtered, placed in cold storage, "aged", transported to the butcher's shop or supermarket and purchased, brought home, stored, prepared and eaten, one can imagine what stage of decay one's dinner is in. According to the Encyclopedia Britannica, body poisons, including uric acid and other toxic wastes are present in the blood and tissue[2].

Meat not only harbours the bacteria infecting the living animal, it may also carry moulds, spores, yeasts and bacilli picked up during post-mortem handling. A book on meat processing explains that the flesh becomes more tender and palatable by the process of ripening, hanging and maturing (ageing). Vic Sussman, in The Vegetarian Alternative (cited in [1]) says "Few meat-eaters would like to hear the words putrefaction, rigor mortis and rotting applied to their sirloin and pot roast. But flesh is flesh though the euphemisms ripening, toughening and enzymatic action are kinder to the ear."

Trained government inspectors use sight, smell and touch in a constant battle to protect meat-eaters from intentional and accidental abuses. But effective regulation of flesh food is enormously difficult. Sussman says (Ibid.) "Even the most conscientious inspectors are forced by circumstances and the pressure of time to let suspect carcasses leave the plant."

Humans who eat the liver's of the animals are bombarded with an even greater concentration of waste products and toxic substances. The liver, being the filtering organ of the body, is loaded with elements the body cannot use, which are trapped in the liver and remain there. Liver eaters are treated to higher concentrations of

15

mercury and artificial hormones, plus other toxic substances which remain in the animal's disposal system (so much for the health benefits of cod liver oil!). Liver increases the amount of creatine in the urine. Creatinuria (abnormal amounts of creatine in the urine) is involved in endocrine (glandular) disorders.

Those who eat processed meats also get many of the odds and ends of the animals: eyes, ears, bladders, lips, udders, snouts and parts of the bones and skin. Not even a meat inspector can tell what part of the body sausages and frankfurters came from - it's all meat tissue and all legal! [1].

Scientific Reports Warning of the Danger of Flesh Eating
Authorities recognise that the basic problem is with the nature of animal flesh itself. For instance, The National Academy of Science reports "Reluctantly, we are forced to recognise the infeasibility of eradicating salmonellosis at this time." ("An evaluation of the Salmonella Problem," National Academy of Sciences, Washington. D.C., cited in [1]).

John A. Scharffenberg, M.D. in *Problems with Meat (1961)*, says "Meat is a major factor in the leading causes of death in the United States and probably in similarly affluent societies. In fact, next to tobacco and alcohol, meat is the greatest single cause of mortality in the United States." He marshals this scientific evidence of the disease potential of meat and the relationship of meat to the following specific problems: atherosclerosis, cancer, decrease in longevity or life expectancy, kidney disorders, osteoporosis, salmonellosis, and trichinosis. He quotes an editorial statement in the Journal of the American Medical Association: "A vegetarian diet can prevent 97% of our coronary occlusions."[1].

Several studies have identified the risk factors of atherosclerosis and heart attacks. For instance, a 1970 study by twenty-nine voluntary health agencies, in co-operation with the American Medical Association (these study groups consisted of many of the nation's top scientists); a 1977 study by the Senate Select Committee on Nutrition and Human Needs: a twelve-year Finnish Mental Hospital Study

16

(Effect of Cholesterol-Lowering Diet on Mortality from Coronary Heart Disease and Other Causes, The Lancet 2:835-38, 1972); and a 1975 study comparing Seventh Day Adventists who had different dietary habits. The Seventh Day Adventist study revealed a 64% vulnerability to coronary heart disease in meat-eaters, 40% for lacto-ovo-vegetarians, and 23% for total vegetarians. The 1977 study by the Senate Select Committee on Nutrition and Human Needs reported the significant deleterious influence of the consumption of dietary cholesterol (animal fat) and recommended the increased use of fruits, vegetables and whole grains, and a decrease in the use of foods containing saturated fat (animal fat)([1]).

Cholesterol is mainly found in animal products. Meat, fish, poultry, dairy products and eggs, etc. all contain cholesterol, while plant products, on the whole, do not. Choosing lean cuts of meat is not enough; the cholesterol is mainly in the lean portion. Many people are surprised to learn that chicken contains as much cholesterol as beef. Every four-ounce serving of beef or chicken contains 100 milligrams of cholesterol. Most shellfish are very high in cholesterol. There is no 'good cholesterol' in any food([6]).

It is worth noting that Eskimos, living largely on meat and fat, age rapidly with an average lifespan of 27½ years. The Kirgese, a nomadic Eastern Russian tribe that live predominantly on meat, mature early and die equally early; they rarely pass the age of 40. In contrast, field investigations of anthropologists of non-meat cultures have documented the radiant health, stamina and longevity enjoyed by people such as the Hunzas of Pakistan, the Otomi Tribe (Natives of Mexico) and Native peoples of the American Southwest. It is not uncommon for such tribes to have healthy and active individuals of 110 years or more. Moreover, diseases such as arthritis, diabetes, cancer, arteriosclerosis, high blood pressure, gallstones, kidney stones, etc. are virtually unheard of in these societies. World Health statistics consistently show that the nations which consume the most meat have the highest incidence of disease (heart disease, cancer) and groups of vegetarians in different countries have the lowest incidence of disease([1]).

17

Reference should also be made to the experiences of Denmark and Norway, where the general health of the people improved when vegetarian diets were adopted during World Wars I and II, including a significant reduction in heart disease. However, both nations reverted to meat diets as soon as the crises passed, and subsequent studies showed that the temporary health advantages had apparently subsided[2].

Indeed, in his book 'The Pritikin Promise'[9], Pritikin recounts the many athletic endurance records held by vegetarians and it is feasible that the endurance prowess is related to the high carbohydrate content of vegetarian food. Dr Douglas Graham, a former U.S. professional trampolinist who has coached top athletes including Martina Navratilova in raw vegan nutrition for optimum athletic performance reports the same thing. He believes that athletes perform better and recover better on a high-fruit and raw vegetable diet. More recent converts of Dr Graham's include the basketball player Ronnie Grandison.

It is not surprising therefore that more recently, plant based and low-fat diets in general have been receiving more attention, and reports are trickling down of medical doctors who are recommending eliminating meat from the diets of arthritis and cancer patients, and even of medical doctors who are acknowledging the health benefits of vegetarianism for themselves and all of their patients. Good and correct information cannot be suppressed forever!

Autopsies performed in Korea showed that 75% of American soldiers had hardened arteries, regardless of their age. Korean soldiers, on a simple diet of vegetables, grains and very little meat, showed essentially no hardening of the arteries.

Animal Diseases
This topic will covered later on in more detail, but for now let us briefly address this issue.

In Dr Parrette's 'Why I Don't Eat Meat' he argues that in a recent Los Angeles Times entitled "Disease Causes Halt of Some Trout Imports."

it is reported that the California Fish and Game Department turned back six tank cars of trout fingerling that were shipped into California to stock lakes and streams, as they were found to be infected with liver cancer[1].

A big danger facing meat eaters is that animals are frequently infected with diseases which are undetected or simply ignored by the meat producers or inspectors. Often, if an animal has cancer or a tumour in a certain part of its body, the cancerous part will be cut away and the rest of the body sold as meat. Or worse yet, the tumours themselves will be incorporated into mixed meats such as hot dogs. In one area of America where there is routine inspection of slaughtered animals, 25,000 cattle with eye cancers were sold as beef. Scientists have found that if the liver of a diseased animal is fed to fish, the fish will get cancer[1].

When one considers the evidence of the cancer-causing potential of meat, it seems incredible that there is no health warning on every package! In addition to cancerous tumours in fowl, there is a carrier form which is impossible to detect except by painstaking laboratory experiments. "The conclusions drawn must consider the possibility that all chickens show the basic microscopic lesions of lymphomatosis." (Dr Eugene F. Oakberg. Poultry Science, May 1950, cited in ([1])).

The rapid rise of leukaemia in cattle calls our attention to the fact that blood cancer, or leukaemia, is now a major cause of death among children in the United States. In fact, meat has been implicated in a wide variety of factors and processes known to be associated with cancer, including the following:

1) Chemical carcinogens, added to the meat, or produced by heating.

2) Cancer viruses found in tumours in animals, which are possibly transmittable to humans.

3) Lessened host resistance to invasive disease.

19

4) The lack of fibre in meat, which increases its transit time through the colon. Adequate fibre is also necessary to help remove bile acids from the gastrointestinal tract. (Colon cancer patients tend to produce more bile acids than other people.)

5) The rapid maturation, earlier menstruation and higher rate of breast cancer amongst meat-eaters.

6) A high-fat diet is also associated with breast cancer.

7) Dr Scharffenberg argues that a meat diet contains high Prolactin levels (Prolactin is a pituitary hormone promoting milk formation and lactation). A high-fat diet increases the Prolactin-Oestrogen ratio, which then enhances mammary tumour growth. When humans change from a meat diet to a vegetarian diet, the Prolactin surge appears to be reduced to almost one half. A diet high in fat, meat and milk tends to increase the incidence of breast cancer. (cited in ([1])).

It has been demonstrated that cancer can be transmitted from one animal species to another. (Relationship of viruses to malignant disease." AMA Arch. Int. Med. 105:482-91, 1960; Canadian Cancer Conf. 4:313-30, 1961; 70 newly recognised viruses in man - Public Health Reports 74:6-12, 1959).

Colon Cancer
Colon cancer is acknowledged to be the predominant type of cancer in the United States, and it is the second leading cause of cancer mortality. An article in the Wall Street Journal several years ago tells about a study of colon cancer by Dr William Haenzel, Dr John W. Berg and others at the National Cancer Institute, as a result of which Dr Berg said, "There is now substantial evidence that beef is a key factor in determining bowel cancer incidence."([1]).

Scientists have reported evidence that two characteristics of meat-based diets are specific influences in colon cancer:

1) Faecal transit time; a low-fibre diet allows carcinogens to be concentrated and held in contact with the bowel mucosa for long periods, while a high residue diet (a vegetarian diet) produces more rapid passage of body waste.

2) Influence of the diet on the amount of carcinogens produced by the body. It has been found that meat fat tends toward production of carcinogens in the intestine.

Diets High in Animal Fat
Dr Ernest L. Wynder, President of the American Health Foundation, and a long-time cancer researcher, reported long ago that the results of his studies had convinced him of the cancer hazards of diets high in animal fats. On 31st March 1982, Dr Wynder, now renowned as the health detective who first linked smoking and cancer a generation ago, reiterated his findings. He said that a low animal fat, high fibre, fresh fruit and vegetable diet helps fight both cancer and heart disease. He said that the American Heart Association and the National Heart, Lung and Blood Institute also recommend such a diet[1].

Dr Anthony B. Miller, Director of the National Cancer Institute of Canada, said: "Evidence suggests that certain foods, particularly high intake of dietary fat, are associated with increased risk of colo-rectal, pancreatic, breast, endometrial, ovarian, prostate and possibly renal cancer." He also recommends increased consumption of fresh fruits and vegetables[1].

Most of the deleterious influences of meat-eating which have been discussed thus far apply to any flesh foods, even those which are raised the "old-fashioned" way, without chemicals or hormones.

Toxic Chemicals in Flesh Foods
In addition, those who eat processed meats are treated to sodium nitrate and sodium nitrite, which together form cancer-causing nitrosamines in the body which are extremely toxic. Sodium nitrate and sodium nitrite are used as preservatives to retard the putrefaction process in processed meats (frankfurters, salami, bologna, sausage,

etc.). These chemicals work by reacting with pigments in the dead animal's blood and muscle (without them, the natural grey-brown colour of the flesh would turn most customers off). The food can still spoil, but it is not as obvious.

In fact, in Consumer Reports (February 1972, pp76) it was reported that after studying samples from thirty-two brands of frankfurters bought in supermarkets throughout the United States, researchers stated: "Food experts generally agree that putrefaction has set in when a frankfurter's total bacteria count has reached ten million per gram. With that as a yardstick, more than forty per cent of the samples we analysed had begun to spoil. One sample tested out at 140 million per gram."

Dr Charles C. Edwards, Commissioner of the Food and Drug Administration, testified before a House Subcommittee in March 1971, stating that sodium nitrite is potentially dangerous to small children, can cause deformities in foetuses, can cause serious damage to anaemic persons and is a possible cause of cancer[1].

The problem is that sodium nitrate and sodium nitrite cannot distinguish between the blood of a corpse and the blood of a living human being and so, when reacting to pigmentation in blood and muscle, many people actually suffer blood poisoning in the process. Even small quantities can prove hazardous. A. J. Lehman of the FDA pointed out that "only a small margin of safety exists between the amount of nitrate that is safe and that which is dangerous"[1].

In fact, Dr Michael Jacobson of the Center for Science in the Public Interest says that sodium nitrate and sodium nitrite in processed meats have caused numerous cases of blood poisoning (methemoglobinemia), many reported in medical journals[1]. He says that meat contains residues of more than a dozen chemicals, which are used to fatten the animals, with each proven to cause cancer. The chemicals and hormones are mixed and administered on the farms by stockmen, who often use greater than recommended amounts, and fail to withdraw drugs far enough ahead of slaughter[1].

Sodium sulphite is used to give meat a fresh, red appearance, even after it has become rancid and turned *black*. This chemical will change it back to bright red, and will also "miraculously" eliminate the strong odour of putrefaction ([1]), of course, one can only imagine the potential hazards for human safety of this chemical!

Both penicillin and tetracycline are routinely used in poultry and cattle feed. When the FDA moved towards restricting the addition to animal feed of antibiotics that are also used to combat human diseases (because of the consequent growth of antibiotic resistant bacteria), the meat industry were outraged at the proposal. Mould can be washed off by the food processors, the meat can be recycled by cutting up, grinding, adding spices, or cooking to disguise colour, odour and taste([1]).

Penman in "The Price of Meat"([3]), argues that although Clenbuterol, which is routinely added to meat, is dangerous to humans its use is widespread. In the six months between October 1992 and March 1993, meat containing Clenbuterol residues killed and hospitalised over 350 in Spain and over 80 people in France (with liver disorders).

Throughout Europe the mild effects of a low level of exposure to Clenbuterol include pulpitations, dizziness and tremors, are thought to have afflicted tens of thousands. A leaked draft report produced by the EU estimated that 80% of Belgians, 60% of Dutch and 25% of British beef cattle are doped with illegal drugs. The use of the cocktails is now accepted by so many farmers that to produce the report the EU had to collect and analyse its own samples from cattle across the continent. Normally they would rely on vets and scientists in each member state, but local vets could be bribed all too easily or threatened to falsify results. In fact, even after it had produced a report, the EU sat on it for nine months for fear of damaging the public's faith in the Meat Industry, eventually releasing a watered-down version perhaps to protect farmers. But even the leaked draft may have under-estimated the problem; farmers, like athletes in training, are learning fast how to mix drug cocktails so that the different chemicals mask each other and confuse the scientists. One senior EU official told the Daily Telegraph in 1993: "I don't eat beef

23

anymore, I used to eat a steak a day. This stuff is not just Clenbuterol - its very dangerous. Some farmers don't know what they've got - they just chuck it in"[3].

Meat animals are treated with many, many chemicals to increase their growth, fatten them quickly, improve their meat colour, etc. In order to produce the most meat at the highest profit, animals are force-fed, injected with hormones to stimulate growth, given appetite stimulants, antibiotics, sedatives and chemical feed mixtures. The New York Times reported: "But of far greater potential danger to the consumer's health are the hidden contaminants - bacteria-like salmonella and residues from the use of pesticides, nitrates, nitrites, hormones, antibiotics and other chemicals" (July 1971). Many of these have been found to be cancer-causing chemicals and, in fact, many animals die of these drugs even before they are led to slaughter. The unnatural practices of meat production not only unbalance the body chemistry of, for instance, chickens and destroy their natural habits, but the growth of malignant tumours and other malformations are quite common results[2].

Drug use, like much of the rest of factory farming, has its roots in post-war posterity, where the only aim was to maximise production and cut prices. The pharmaceutical industry was quick to spot a potential market; the first successful product was diethylstilbestrol (DES), which was injected into an animal's muscles and made it grow rapidly. But that, too, came at a price: It was a possible carcinogen and several countries banned its use. In fact, according to G. and S. Null (cited in [4]) DES, which has been used in the US for at least the last 20 years (possibly because the FDA estimate that it saves meat produces more than $500 million annually), has been shown in studies to be carcinogenic and has been banned as a serious health hazard in 32 different countries. By the 1980s, it had been suspected of inducing breast growth in baby boys and the early signs of puberty in Italian girls of less than a year old: the children's symptoms were linked to DES residues in certain meat-based baby foods. Other symptoms of DES poisoning have included endometriosis, uterine disorders, cancer of the reproductive organs and breasts, etc. Traces of

DES were found in U.S. meat even as late as late 1999, even though its banned([7]).

Another popular growth stimulant is arsenic! In 1972, this substance was found by the USDA (US Department of Agriculture) to exceed the legal limit in 15% of the nation's poultry([4]).

In 1988, a range of growth-promoting drugs were banned in the EU; only Britain voted against the resolution. By 1994, meat exports from the US plummeted from USD 231M in 1988 to USD 98M and the US is now threatening to take action against the EU through the WHO because it is probably illegal to ban hormone treated meat from entering Europe. And, needless to say, the pharmaceutical industry, sensing vast profits, wants the ban lifted([3]).

The ban is controversial because it blocks the use of all growth-promoters, several of which have passed the licensing producers in some European countries, as well as in the USA, Canada and Latin America. The EU's own scientific studies, commissioned before the ban was imposed in 1988, found that three 'natural' hormones, oestradiol beta-17, progesterone and testosterone, were not a threat to consumers, if used properly. In late 1995, the US case was reinforced when Codex, the international food standards body of the United Nation's Food and Agricultural Organisation and the World Health Organisation (WHO), signified its approval of the five hormones used in the USA (Ibid.).

There are also dangerous levels of dioxin in meat from all the industrialised countries, according to the EU's Scientific and Veterinary Committee. The danger comes from grazing land close to industrial plants and incinerators. About 1% of meat production exceeds the permitted levels of this deadly pollution, following revelations of lavatory, animal and oil waste sludge in fodder which lead to a different dioxin scare across Europe (Ibid.).

Regarding pesticides, you should note that eating low on the food chain significantly reduces the threat of pesticide residues. Tests in Britain have shown the pesticide residue levels to be highest in meat-eaters, lower in lacto-vegetarians, and lowest in total vegetarians. This is due to the concentrating factor as the contaminant goes through the additional link in the ecological chain and the animal concentrates the pollutant in its body. *The meat-eater may eat in a few minutes the pesticides that an animal has accumulated over a lifetime.*

All over the world, fields are being treated with poisonous chemicals (fertilisers and pesticides). These poisons are retained in the bodies of the animals that eat the plants and grasses. For instance, fields are sprayed with the insect-killing chemical DDT, a very powerful poison which scientists say can cause cancer, sterility and serious liver disease. DDT and pesticides like it are retained in animal fat and, once stored, are difficult to break down. Thus, as cows eat grass or feed, whatever pesticides they eat are mostly retained so that when you eat meat you are taking into your body all the concentrations of DDT and other chemicals that have accumulated during the animal's lifetime. Thus you are the final consumer and the recipient of the highest concentration of poisonous pesticides - meat contains approximately 13 times as much DDT as vegetables, fruits and grass. Iowa State University performed experiments which showed that most of the DDT in human bodies comes from meat[2]. In fact, according to the Life Science Institute, **pesticide residues are 16 to several hundred times higher in meat and milk products than in fresh fruit and vegetables!**

In fact, a study by the Washington DC based Environmental Defense Fund revealed that breast milk of vegetarian women contained significantly lower levels of pesticide residues than that of meat-eating women. Further, research by author Nat Altman disclosed that vegetables and nuts contain about 1/7 the pesticide residues of flesh foods: fruits and legumes about 1/8 as much; and grains about 1/24 as much[1].

The fact is that it is much more difficult to have even a reasonably good diet with meat than without it. In the first place, even the much vaunted "complete protein" status of meat is, at best, based on a colossal error. The complete protein of the animal could exist only if the animal were consumed raw and whole. Meat-eating animals eat the blood, bones, cartilage's, liver, etc. of their prey - not just the muscle and fat. They eat it raw and do not lose any of the mineral elements. Therefore, muscle meat (most commonly consumed by humans) serves as grossly inadequate as a protein source. On the other hand, humans who eat the livers of the animals don't win either. As previously indicated, those who eat liver are exposed to greater concentrations of morbid substances. Even though liver is touted as an optimal source of such substances as iron, Vitamin A and Vitamin B12, it can hardly be regarded as anything remotely resembling wholesome food([1]).

For years, conventional nutritionists have maintained that complete and optimal nutrition is assured on a diet using animal foods as the primary source of protein, and that a vegetarian diet presents many problems. Dr Scharffenberg produces well-documented scientific evidence (Ibid.) indicating that, in fact, the truth is exactly the opposite. He argues that **cooked muscle meat is deficient in vitamins, minerals, fibre and carbohydrates and excessively high in fat and concentrated protein.**

Meat is one of the main sources of food that provide little fibre. In fact, *flesh foods lengthen the average transit time through the gastrointestinal tract from thirty hours to seventy-seven hours.* Meat contains virtually no carbohydrates and is excessively high in fat and concentrated protein. Dr Bircher-Benner, the great Swiss physician, said that meat does not give strength and that is lacks certain minerals and vitamins and introduces too much fat and protein into the system, disturbing the balance of nutrition and giving rise to intestinal putrefaction (Ibid.).

Hereward Carrington, (cited in [1]) argues that meat is a highly *stimulating* article of food, and for that reason it is innutritious. He argues that stimulation and nutrition invariably exist in inverse ratio - one to the other, and vice versa. The very fact that meat is a stimulant, as is now universally conceded to be, shows us that it is more or less an innutritious article of diet and that it contains poisonous elements and that the supposed "strength" we receive from the meat is due entirely to the stimulating effects upon the system of the various poisons, or toxic substances, introduced into the system, together with the meat. It is for this reason that those who leave off meat experience a feeling of lassitude and weakness in the first few days - they lack the stimulation formerly supplied, and now notice the reaction which invariably follows such stimulation. This feeling of weakness or "all-goneness" is therefore to be expected and is in no way proof that the diet is weakening the person. If they persist in their reformed manner of living for some time, they will find that this reaction wears off and that a general and continued feeling of energy and well-being will follow.

The tremendous amounts of protein frequently recommended, namely 75 to 100 grams daily (or more) are far in excess of the body's needs and are the source of much trouble. The famous nutritionists Dr Ragnar Berg, Dr R. Chittenden, Dr M. Hindehede, Dr M. Hegsted, Dr C. Rose and others have shown in extensive experiments that our actual need for protein is somewhere around thirty grams a day, or even less. Many leading contemporary scientists and nutritionists in Europe, such as Dr Ralph Bircher, Dr Bircher-Benner, Dr Otto Buchinger Jr., Dr H. Karstrom, Prof. H. A. Schweigart and many others are in full agreement with the findings of Drs. Berg, Chittenden, Rose et al. and are recommending a low protein diet as the diet most conducive to good health([1]).

High Incidence of Degenerative Diseases
The Seventh-Day Adventists and Mormons, who advocate a low animal-protein diet, have fifty to seventy per cent lower death rates than those of average Americans. They also are reported to have a much lower incidence of cancer, tuberculosis, coronary diseases, blood and kidney disease, and diseases of the digestive and respiratory organs.

Negative Lime Balance (Calcium Transfer):
Bone calcium is at dangerously low levels in those using meat as compared to vegetarians, especially in people over fifty. A high-protein (especially meat protein) diet increases the urinary excretion of calcium. Thus vegetarians are less prone to osteoporosis (porous bones) (see chapter on Osteoporosis). H. J. Curtis in a book entitled

28

Biological Mechanism of Ageing gives supporting evidence to the theory of animal protein causing osteoporosis. Calcium is transferred from the hard tissues (bones) to the soft tissues (arteries, skin, joints, internal organs and eyes). Transfer of calcium to the soft tissues results in catastrophic fractures, hardening of the arteries, wrinkling of skin, arthritis, the formation of stones, cataracts, high blood pressure, degeneration of internal organs, loss of hearing, senility and cancer (Ibid.).

Athletes who eat much meat are especially susceptible to arthrosis, a degenerative process of the joints. Among twenty conventional-diet professional football players who were observed for eighteen years, 100% suffered ankle arthrosis and 97. 5% suffered knee arthrosis. A negative lime balance is easily produced by increased protein supply, as we will see later. The eminently important minerals - potassium and magnesium - are known to be deficient in an every day diet rich in meat, eggs, cheese, fat, sugar and grains, but richly present in a full-value vegan diet predominating in raw food (Ibid.).

Animals who live on a predominantly meat-based diet usually have an accelerated growth rate which equals accelerated maturity, accelerated degeneration and accelerated demise. Rapid growth and short life go together, verified by repeated studies and experiments. Since rapid maturation occurs as a result of high protein diets, this produces earlier onset of menstruation (Ibid.).

It must be emphasised that diet alone is not the single component in cancer and other degenerative diseases, but optimal nutrition does play a fundamental and preventive role, and faulty dietary habits play a causative role.

Kofranyi of the Nlax Planck Institute in Russia proved that complete nitrogen balance and performance ability could be maintained on 25 grams of protein daily, and Oomen and Hipsley found a population that develops not just full health, but magnificent structure and corresponding physical performance on 15 to 20 grams of protein daily[1].

Sherman, a member of the American Research Council's Food and Nutrition Board who agree on daily requirement for different food elements, argues that evidence points toward a much lower amount being required, somewhere around thirty-five grams. However, if the protein requirement had been set so low, there would have been a public outcry, so a corresponding "margin of safety" was adopted, and "seventy grams" was published. Because the scientific basis for this was non-existent, the word "recommendation" was used instead of "requirement". Of course, it was publicly interpreted as the requirement, in fact, as the minimum (Ibid.).

"The smallest amount of food able to keep the body in a state of high efficiency is physiologically the most economical, and thus best adapted for the body's needs." This is the Chittenden concept, stated years ago by Russell Henry Chittenden, which applies forcibly to protein. The average American diet contains 45% more protein than even the National Academy of Sciences recommends and is certainly not "best adapted for the body's needs."[5].

Let us now examine the charge that flesh-eating is supposed to be a superior source of protein. Well, upon examining the evidence, the truth is exactly opposite! The effects of encumbering our bodies with the proteins of other animals serves to promote diseased conditions of the human organism. Dr Herbert M. Shelton says that allergy and anaphylaxis (a kind of toxic shock of the tissues) are not mysterious and that they are due to long-standing poisoning of the body by excess or inappropriate protein foods. Animal proteins are often not reduced to their constituent amino acids, but are absorbed in more complex form. Absorption by the body of such partially digested proteins poisons the human body and so-called "allergic symptoms" may result in gout, arthritis, cancer, or any one or more of a host of degenerative diseases[1].

A meat-eater must also be concerned about digestive problems caused by too little dietary fibre; circulatory problems due to excessive cholesterol deposits from animal fats; loss of bone mass due to inadequate ingestion and retention of calcium; deficiency of vitamins and minerals; and inadequate carbohydrate intake (without increasing calories)([1]).

The Erroneous Amino Acid Theory
One of the favourite arguments of flesh-eaters is that proteins from the plant kingdom are "incomplete," because, they say, no plant food contains all of the twenty-three identical amino acids. Studies of man's physiology and the effect of his consumption of foods from plant kingdom have shown conclusively that it is not necessary to consume all of the amino acids at one sitting, or even the eight (some references say ten) "essential" amino acids that are not fabricated within the body. Foods we eat are processed by the body, and the amino acids, vitamins and minerals, and other nutrients reserved in a pool for later use as needed. When we eat, we replenish the reserves in this pool, which is then drawn upon by cells as and when required. We do not live upon one protein food, but upon the protein content of our varied diet, which provides all of the protein needs of the body. Guyton's "Guidance Textbook of Medical Physiology" is authority to this important information. The book shows that amino acids are picked up from the bloodstream and cells of the body.

Nowhere in nature is there any evidence of the necessity for such complicated manoeuvering to obtain optimal nutrition. Not only are humans not dependent on the animal kingdom for their nutrition, it is also not necessary to a numbers game with nutrients or foods at each meal. The intelligently planned meatless diet has none of the disease problems of flesh foods and provides a dependable source of all the nutrients - including adequate protein. Complex judgements or computations, such as those in planning a meat-based diet, are obviated. It is extremely difficult for meat-eaters to maintain a diet low in saturated fat and cholesterol, high in carbohydrates and fibre and containing adequate calcium to compensate for effects of including meat in their diet.

Hence, new knowledge has completely reversed the old theory, which was based on studies between 1929 and 1930 and used purified amino acids. We do not eat purified amino acids. Recurring studies reported in the *Journal of the American Medical Association* and other

31

medical journals in 1950 show that it is not necessary to feed complete protein at each meal. One such study by E. S. Nasset, reported in *'World Review of Nutrition and Dietetics'* (1972, pp134-153) indicated that the body can make up any of the amino acids missing in a particular meal from its amino acid pool of reserves, as long as a variety of foods are provided in the diet.

Dr Scharffenberg states that vegetable protein is not lacking totally in any specific amino acid and that an average vegetarian ingests adequate amounts of protein. He argues that the amount of essential amino acids in the diet not only meet the minimum requirement, they more than twice exceed them (cited in [1]). It is true that protein is not stored in the body in the same sense that excess carbohydrates are stored as glycogen or fat, but the body can compensate for temporary deficiencies, by withdrawing what it needs from the pool of materials within the organism (the amino acid pool), as material is sloughed off intestinal walls from digestive secretions, and from the autolysis of old cells, fat, etc. Many foods from the plant kingdom contain so-called "complete" proteins; that is, humans may obtain from them all of the essential amino acids which they cannot synthesise, but from which other amino acids may be synthesised as needed. Moreover, cooked and coagulated animal protein presents great difficulties in the necessary breakdown of the long chains of amino acids of meat and results in not only inevitable putrefaction, but a grave loss of vital energy[1].

Nuts are a good source of raw protein-rich food. All nuts, except the hickory, contain complete proteins. This has been verified by experiments by Cajori, Kellogg and Berg. Sunflower seeds and sesame seeds are in the same category. Peanuts, beans and a long list of vegetables also contain all the essential amino acids as well as carrots, Brussels sprouts, cabbage, cauliflower, collard greens, fresh corn, cucumbers, eggplant, kale, okra, peas, potatoes, summer squash, sweet potatoes and tomatoes. (This listing is by no means complete.) Most vegetables, of course, contain lesser amounts of amino acids than do concentrated proteins like nuts, seeds and legumes which is not a bad thing! For adequate protein supplies, use a variety of the available natural foods - choosing from fruits, vegetables, nuts, seeds and sprouts, not all at each meal of course, or even necessarily every day, but over the course of the weekly diet (Ibid.).

Dr Hoobler, researching at Yale University, demonstrated the superiority of nut protein. It was he who proved conclusively that the protein of nuts not only provides greater nutritive efficiency than that of meat, milk and eggs, but that it is also more effective than a combination of these three animal proteins. Fruits and vegetables, though containing relatively smaller amounts of protein in their natural state, are excellent sources of supplementary amino acids for complete and optimal nutrition (Ibid.). The protein in raw nuts and seeds, and in uncooked fruits and vegetables, are readily available to the body, and are therefore said to be of high biological value. During the process of digestion, the long chains of amino acids (the building blocks of protein) are gradually broken up for the body's use in synthesising its own protein (as any species must do). However, when proteins have been cooked or preserved, they are coagulated. Enzyme resistant linkages are formed which resist cleavage, and the amino acids may not be released for body use. In this case, the protein is useless and/or poisonous to the body, becoming soil for bacteria and a poisonous decomposition by-product (Ibid.).

Since the nutrients available from raw food are several hundred per cent greater than those available from food that has been cooked or otherwise processed, and since flesh foods are usually not eaten raw and whole by humans, this in itself would be an important reason why first-hand protein foods from the plant kingdom, which may be eaten uncooked, are superior (Ibid.).

CONCLUSION

In this chapter we have reversed many myths about flesh foods. We have learned about the unsuitability to our physiology of a flesh-based diet and learned of the various toxins which in one way or other enter our bodies when we consume flesh foods. Moreover, we have learned of some of the diseases which farm animals are increasingly suffering from, which makes meat an increasingly undesirable option!

33

Below then is a summary of the specific health reasons for eliminating flesh foods from the diet:-

1) Flesh foods cause putrefaction by decomposing in the intestines, reducing the functioning of intestinal flora, and interfering with the synthesis and utilisation of Vitamin B12.

2) The by-products of toxic substances (uric acid, purines, etc.) and carcinogens cause degenerative diseases.

3) Saturated fats from meat produce abnormal cholesterol deposits, causing heart and arterial degeneration.

4) Meats contain parasites, chemicals and hormones, which damage the body and cause disease.

5) Diseased animals can pass their diseases on to humans.

6) Flesh foods provide a favourable medium for the multiplication of the bacteria of disease.

7) Flesh foods lessen the resistance of the body to disease.

8) Meat-based diets present complex and grave nutritional problems.

9) People who eliminate meat from their diets are better nourished and have better health and greater longevity than meat-eaters.

We will now go on to address some more myths about the consumption of flesh foods in the rest of this section, and consequently in the rest of this book.

CHAPTER TWO: THE VITAMIN B12 ISSUE

Some people have been told that if they consume a diet which does not include animal products they will be deficient in vitamin B12 and will become victims of pernicious anaemia. The medical profession and the meat industry are guilty of propagating this type of misinformation! However, if we think logically we may ask ourselves: If meat contains vitamin B12, where does the herbivorous cow get this vitamin from? The truth is that vitamin B12 is manufactured by the friendly bacteria in the animal's intestinal tract. This is true for all vegetarian animals, whether herbivores or frugivores, including human beings.

Although many people argue that the only foods which contain vitamin B12 are animal-derived foods, this is untrue. No foods naturally contain vitamin B12 - neither animal or plant foods. Vitamin B12 is a microbe - a bacteria - it is produced by microorganisms. B12 synthesis is known to occur naturally in the human small intestine (in the ileum), which is the primary site of B12 absorption. As long as gut bacteria have cobalt and certain other nutrients, they produce vitamin B12. Without organic cobalt, the human body cannot manufacture vitamin B12.

A vitamin B12 deficiency is a serious disorder, but it is never just a B12 deficiency because vitamin and mineral deficiencies never happen in isolation. Indications of a deficiency of vitamin B12, when they do reach a stage where they have shown up, can be quite severe. Fatigue, paleness, anorexia, mental confusion, delusions, paranoia, weight loss, pernicious anaemia (a shortfull of red blood cells), menstrual problems, tremors and listlessness, are just some indications that a person may have a B12-deficiency.

UK official recommendations have decreased in recent years, the body's needs having been previously over-estimated. Indeed, the Department of Health recognises that some people have lower than average requirements of B12. A whole lifetime's requirement of B12 add up to a 40 milligram speck of red crystals, about one-seventh the size of an average tablet of aspirin! Taking large doses of the vitamin by mouth is pointless because 3ug is the most that can be absorbed at any one time([9]).

Vitamin B12 is excreted in the bile and is effectively reabsorbed. This is known as enterohepatic circulation. The amount of B12 excreted in the bile can vary from 1 to 10ug (micrograms) a day. People on diets low in B12, including vegans and some vegetarians, may be obtaining more B12 from reabsorption than from dietary sources. Reabsorption is the reason it can take over 20 years for a deficiency disease to develop. In comparison, if B12 deficiency is due to a failure in absorption, it can take only three years for a deficiency disease to occur ([10]).

A deficiency of Vitamin B12, which is a forerunner of pernicious anaemia, is not necessarily due to dietary inadequacy. Indeed, a report released from a Vitamin B12 Conference stated, "Pernicious anaemia appears to arise not from a shortage in the diet, but from impairment of the ability to absorb Vitamin B12." (cited in ([1])). In fact, study after study has shown that the deficiency of vitamin B12 is often due to the lack of absorption of the vitamin from the intestinal tract, due to the absence of "intrinsic factor," a substance which is normally present in the gastric juices.

Putrefactive bacteria can destroy friendly bacteria thus inhibiting the synthesis and absorption of Vitamin B12. The principal cause of putrefaction in the human digestive tract is the ingestion of cooked animal protein (though putrefaction can occur as a result of bad food combining or overeating of any concentrated protein foods).

According to Dr Gabriel Cousens([20]), even if a blood test does reveal that you are low in vitamin B12, this may not mean that you are deficient because, if you are on a healthy raw-food diet for instance, you actually require less of this vitamin. Low serum B12 levels do not equate to a B12 deficiency necessarily. A low level of vitamin B12 in the bloodstream does not mean that there is a deficiency in the body as a whole, it may well be being utilised by the living cells (such as the central nervous system). In any case, a person who takes supplements may well have 'vitamin B12' floating in their bloodstream, but this does not mean it is usable to the human body. Serum (blood) tests are, anyhow, less reliable than urine tests.

Nevertheless, when a person does have a vitamin B12 deficiency this is certainly not a condition which cannot be remedied. The best thing one can do is to consult with a natural hygienic professional and to consider a fast (which should be supervised by a qualified fasting supervisor - for more information, contact the author). Dr Vetrano, an American hygienic practitioner of many years standing argues that there have been repeated instances of improvement in the condition of the blood as a result of fasting, plus subsequent improvement in the diet, especially when flesh foods are eliminated[2].

The myth that plants do not contain B12 has been propagated and fostered by vested interests. The truth is that B12 is found in plants in very small amounts. This is consistent with the fact that our need for Vitamin B12 is minuscule (under one microgram (a millionth of a gram) daily, and the body can store it for two to eight years (Vitamins of the B Complex, 1959 U.S. Department of Agriculture Yearbook of Agriculture, Section on Food, pp139-149). Vitamin B12 has been found in significant amounts in many plant foods, some of which are bananas, dates, greens, peanuts, and particularly sprouts and raw sunflower seeds[1].

A correspondent to the *New England Journal of Medicine* (cited in [1]) notes that vitamin B12 is manufactured by micro-organisms, making it possible to obtain B12 from certain seeds and nuts, and from soya beans (please note that cooked soya beans will lose their B vitamins quickly since vitamin B is a water-soluble vitamin and that raw, even sprouted soya beans may contain toxic substances). The correspondent also cites synthesis of the vitamin in the digestive tract of humans when adequate amounts of unheated seeds are eaten, and points to healthy babies who are breast-fed by strict vegetarian mothers. Furthermore, from studies of vegetarians, Dr Wolfgang Tiling discovered the synthesis of B12 in the intestines of children on a soya milk diet.

More recent research at the Loma Linda University found excellent B12 levels for tested vegans (people who eat plant foods only) who eat all, or most of their food fresh and unheated. Vitamin B12 is water soluble, and therefore best obtained in raw foods (Ibid.). Studies have demonstrated that vitamin B12 is heat-sensitive and normal cooking can destroy as much as 89% of it. Indeed, Dr Gabriel Cousens argues that more recent studies have suggested that up to 96% of the B12 can be destroyed by cooking.

High consumption of fat and protein, refined foods and tobacco increase the need for vitamin B12, while at the same time interfering with the synthesis and absorption of this vitamin. Thus, the conventional meat-eater is indeed a more likely candidate for Vitamin B12 deficiency and pernicious anaemia than the individual on an adequate vegetarian diet([1]). It is interesting to note that a study just completed by the USDA found that the vitamin B12 in meat, fish and poultry - while plentiful - is so poorly absorbed in some humans that it leads to B12 deficiency in 9% of the study population of American adults age 26-83 and in another 39% of the group the B12 level was in the "low-normal" range. In other words, almost half of this normal American group had sub-optimal B12 levels despite eating plenty of foods commonly recommended as good B12 sources([17]).

Known as the energy vitamin, not all vitamin B12 functions are clear yet according to very recent vitamin books in the UK. This vitamin may be indirectly important in the production of neurotransmitters in the brain such as dopamine and seratonin which affect moods, sleep patterns, memory and other psychological and physiological functions. Vitamin B12 is involved in creating nerve coverings called myelin sheath, it supports growth, appetite and red blood cell production; it also affects our weight and nervous system. I believe that ME is a B12-deficiency disorder. If you do think you may have a B12-deficiency, it would be wise for you to seek the advice of a health practitioner (such as myself) who is knowledgeable about B12-deficiencies, for immediate advice. This disorder can eventually lead to death if left unchecked.

Since vitamin B12 is recycled in a healthy body, in principle, internal B12 synthesis could fulfil our needs without any B12 provided in the diet, but if cobalt is lacking in our diet, the problem is not so much a lack of B12 synthesising intestinal flora, as a lack of cobalt (which again will need other factors for efficient absorption). This is because vitamin B12 is the only vitamin that contains a trace element - cobalt - which gives this vitamin its chemical name - cobalamin. Cobalt is at the centre of its molecular structure. Humans and all vertebrates require cobalt, although it is assimilated only in the form of vitamin B12. Recent research reveals that in Britain deficiencies are usually due to pernicious anaemia caused by impaired uptake or transport of vitamin B12.

Among the many controversies surrounding vitamin B12, there is the argument that, although intrinsic factor is produced in our stomachs and that our intestines are known to produce vitamin B12, the bacteria is produced too low down in the intestines and cannot be absorbed by our bodies. This argument is sadly still hanging around, however, according to Dr Vetrano, it was disproved by research over 20 years ago([1]). It is nothing more than an obsolete scientific theory. Indeed, in a 1999 version of 'Human Anatomy and Physiology' by Marieb([6]), it states quite clearly that we do indeed absorb vitamin B12 through our intestines.

According to Dr Michael Klaper, vitamin B12 is present in the mouth and intestines. B12 must be combined with a mucoprotein enzyme named Intrinsic Factor, which is normally present in gastric secretions, to be properly assimilated. If the intrinsic factor is impaired or absent, B12 synthesis will not take place, no matter how much is present in the diet([18]).

Factors adversely affecting B12 levels include antibiotics (also contained in milk), alcohol (alcohol damages the liver, so drinkers need more B12), smoking (and all high temp cooked food is smoky), stress, Crohn's disease, drugs/ulcer medication, gastric surgery, genetic predisposition, heavy metals (e.g. mercury), lack of intrinsic factor, prolonged iron deficiency, tapeworm infestation and oral contraceptives. Also, there may be a relationship with vitamin B12 and tinnusitis, multiple sclerosis, Alzheimer's disease, cardiovascular disease, AIDS and neural tube defects([13,14]).

Until recently, algae and other commercially available seaweeds (including spirulina) were touted as containing large amounts of vitamin B12, but they have now been proven to be a B12-antagonist - they actually prevents the absorption of vitamin B12([10]). However, in very up-to-date studies it has been shown that raw nori does in fact contain vitamin B12, but it is of course difficult to obtain raw nori and nori as well as other sea vegetables will inevitably contain poisonous sea salt.

According to 'The Vitamin Bible', vitamin B1 and B2 deficiencies mask vitamin B12 deficiences. Also, folate protects against the anaemia of vitamin B12 deficiency but not the neurological symptoms which can be misleading in connection with victims of pernicious anaemia since vegetarian and vegan diets contain high amounts of folic acid. In fact, intakes of 1mg per day or more of folic acid mask the symptoms of pernicious anaemia.

A major problem in this issue is that many nutritional analyses of foodstuffs were carried out a long time ago, and, as such, have not taken account of more up-to-date technology in scientific procedures. Indeed, according to Dr Vetrano, current books on nutrition in the U.S. have now stated that there is B12 in any food that contains quantities of the B vitamin complex, but previously they were just not able to assay the amounts[7]. Nowadays, more modern technology has allowed them to discover that there is B12 in those foods rich in the B complex. According to the Hutchinson's Almanac 2001, soya beans are a form of cyanocobolamin.

Research in 1992 and 1994 concluded that vitamin B12 found on the leaves and seeds of plants was absorbed by the plant from the soil rather than simple surface contamination. Soil concentrations differ widely and different levels are reported in different plants which may be the result of inaccurate methods of testing the vitamin B12 levels[11].

Vitamin B12 deficiency is not more widespread in vegans or vegetarians - this is just another meat and dairy marketing lie! In fact, many so-called studies 'showing vegans deficient' have to be carefully studies themselves - many of them do not prove vegans to be deficient at all! Contrary to meat and dairy industry propaganda, meat-eaters are known to be more likely to have a vitamin B12 deficiency - this has been known since 1959[2]! According to Dr Bruce Berkowsky, the overwhelming majority of B12 deficiency cases occur amongst the flesh-eating population[21]. The trouble is that once we have damaged our intestinal flora, it is difficult to correct without proper and knowledgeable healthcare and dietary advice. It is of far greater importance to correct intestinal flora problems than to rely on so-called supplements. People who have a physical problem because they think they are not getting enough vitamin B12 are simply not assimilating their foods properly because of poor digestion. When digestion is straightened out, B12 can be utilised and produced once again.

According to Marieb's 'Human Anatomy and Physiology', vitamin B12 can be destroyed by highly alkaline and highly acid conditions. It follows therefore that the B12 in meat would be easily destroyed because the hydrochloric acid in our stomachs during the digestion of meat is highly acidic. This may explain why meat-eaters are so likely to have a B12 deficiency - even though their diet contains vitamin B12. Also, for meat-eaters, there is antibiotics contained in meat! Of course, many meat-eaters destroy their friendly bacteria in their intestines by constant putrefaction and the putrefactive bacteria naturally present in meat will give the body a hard time.

Commercially, vitamin B12 tablets are made from bacteria and the bacteria is deeply fermented. A healthy body will usually expel fermented substances. The main problem with supplement tablets is that they:

1)   Do not contain the hundreds of other nutrients we may need to be healthy that raw foods provide.
2)   They contain artificial substances/contaminants that are detrimental to health.
3)   They are isolated nutrients and as such will not provide for the needs of the body as vitamins and minerals work synergistically.

According to Dr. John Potter PhD, of Fred Hutchinson Cancer Center, Seattle, "Food's magic is based on thousands of complex interactions of dozens of different phytochemicals which are difficult to recreate in pills. While 190 solid studies prove that fruit and vegetables benefit, supplements have only a smattering of evidence". Vitamins, minerals, hormones, etc. do not work in isolation, they work symbiotically. They work with other nutrients in order for their work to be carried out. When these highly complex substances are disturbed, their overall effectiveness can be reduced. However, too much of a nutrient is draining on our vital energy as the human (or non-human) organism may have to expel a nutrient overload. Also, it is doubtful whether, even if you do have a B12 deficiency, you have only a B12 deficiency. A healthier diet and living conditions, as well as a fast, may be in order.

According to Dr Douglas Graham, in his book 'Nutrition and Athletic Performance'([4]), supplementation has proven to be an inadequate and incomplete method of supplying nutrients as scientists cannot match nature's refined balances. He says that since an estimated ninety per cent of all

41

nutrients are as yet undiscovered, why would we want to start adding nutrients into our diet one at a time rather than eating whole foods? Most nutrients are known to interact symbiotically with at least eight other nutrients and considering this, the odds of healthfully supplying any nutrients in its necessary component package becomes 'infinitesimally minute'. More to the point he adds, 'there has never been a successful attempt to keep an animal or human healthy, or even alive, on a diet composed strictly of nutritional supplements'.

Dan Reeter, at Bio-Systems Laboratories in Colorado is creating one of the world's most comprehensive computer facilities for soil biology testing. He says that, from his extensive tests, plants grown in organically managed soil make significantly higher levels of usable vitamin B12. It has also been reported that vitamin B12 is present in wild fruits and wild and home-grown plant foods.

The author contends that animal and dairy produce are a poor source of Vitamin B12 since the vitamin is contained in nutrient-deranged foodstuffs which will inevitably destroy the usability of the vitamin. Indeed, Dr David Ryde argues that in his 45 years of medical practice, all the B12 deficiencies he has witnessed have occurred in meat-eaters([23]). Studies show that those following a typical animal-based diet require more vitamin B12 than those who do not. This is because the typical diet leads to digestive atrophy. Because B12 is peptide-bound in animal products and must be enzymatically cleaved from the peptide bonds to be absorbed, a weakened gastric acid and gastric enzyme secretions (due to a cooked food diet) causes an inability to efficiently extract vitamin B12 from external food. Nevertheless, raw food vegans who have a more powerful digestion actually get more B12 by reabsorption from the bile than they do from external food. Wolfe argues that the natural soil microbes and bacteria found on wild plant foods and unwashed garden plants are typically adequate to supply our B12 requirements. The natural microbes in the soil need to be duplicated and to colonise in our digestive tract, without fermentation or putrefaction.

Another point worth considering is that vitamin B12 Recommended Daily Allowances (RDA's) are based upon the average cooked food ('meat and two veg'), smoking, drinking person. Since meat-eaters are known to require twice the amount of vitamin B12 than a person on a healthier diet, commercial interests have indeed grossly exaggerated our needs for many nutrients. These studies tell us nothing of the requirements for a healthy vegetarian. It is very difficult to determine precise individual needs of any vitamin or nutrient, and an overload of any vitamin or other nutrient creates an unnecessary burden on our vital domain. Factors such as rate of metabolism, stress, etc. can determine our differing and often changing needs. Dr Victor Herbert reported in the American Journal of Clinical Nutrition (1998, Volume 48) that only 0.00000035 ounces (1 microgram) of vitamin B12 is required per day. These minimum vitamin requirements may be inadequate to explain the needs of a healthy raw food vegan, for example, who may require less B12 due to an improved gastric ability and a high ability to recycle vitamin B12. (Cooking destroys microbes and a highly sterilised, cooked vegan diet may not provide the intestines with enough good quality flora). Absorption rates of B12 are higher in healthy individuals than in unhealthy individuals. Indeed, studies based on healthy Indian vegetarian villagers showed that none of them exhibited symptoms of B12 deficiency, despite levels of .3-.5 micrograms of B12[20].

Annie and Dr David Jubb argue that people have lived in such a sterile, antiseptic environment for so long that these necessary symbiotic organisms have been less than present in our diet. They argue that by ingesting soil-born organisms you can maintain an enormous reservoir of uncoded antibodies ready to transform specific pathogens, the way nature intended - by eating a little dirt![8]

Harvey Diamond argues that the entire nutrient issue has been made so confusing with contradictory information that it is no wonder that people are bewildered about where to obtain sufficient nutrients[2]. Unfortunately, some people have been so totally misguided and scared that no amount of common-sense reasoning of even factual data can rescue them from the meat, dairy and petrochemical (synthetic food 'supplement' suppliers) multi-million pound industries. The truth is that whatever nutrients the body needs will be contained in its natural foods (for human beings, raw plant foods). Mother Nature knows how to provide for her own. Why would it be that we are created in such a way as to make us a natural plant-eater and hey presto, there is no vitamin B12 provided for us by plants? If you can't get it from raw fruits, vegetables, nuts, seeds or sprouts then WE DON'T NEED IT! Just because a wild fruit or organic foodstuff contains only a small amount, this does not mean it is deficient. It means that we only need a small amount!

The pill pushers are quick to say that our soil is deficient, but according to Diamond and others, if a seed does not receive the elements it needs IT WILL NOT GROW (OR WILL GROW POORLY - author). Also, plants obtain nutrients from other sources in greater amounts: the sun, water and the air. Plants actually obtain only about 1% of nutrients from the soil[2].

If you do develop a B12 deficiency, certain urgent dietary adjustments may need to be made, and there is a possibility that fasting is in order. You would be well-advised to seek the services of a competent hygienic practitioner whereby certain dietary adjustments may take place and a fast may well be advised.

Upon switching to a healthier diet, be it vegetarian, vegan or raw food (for optimum health), we should go back to nature as much as possible and pay little attention to germ phobics who advise us to scrub our vegetables and fruits. Buy organic and eat home-grown or wild foods and do not clean them too scrupulously! Just as nature intended!.

To summarise then, if a person is healthy and on a healthy vegan, high-percentage raw food diet and does not habitually over-eat, wrongly combine their foods or abuse their bodies generally, and utilises fasting on occasion, it is far less likely that they will develop B12 deficiency symptoms, providing their intestinal flora was not previously deranged. Breast-feeding is an important factor here too, as studies have shown that babies who have been breast-fed are less likely to develop deficiency problems with this vitamin.

Vitamin B12 deficiency is usually symptomatic of a larger problem i.e. poor intestinal flora, poor absorption and also lack of sunlight. It is clear that, on a predominantly raw food, plant-based diet our bodies should be taking in all the essential vitamins and minerals it needs. However, as mentioned earlier, assimilation and absorption by the body may be a problem, in which case fasting is the answer and then a high raw food diet should be adopted.

Please note that it is not recommended for anyone to go on a fast of longer duration than 1½ days without competent fasting supervision, as prolonged fasts can lead to serious detoxification symptoms and must be monitored by a qualified fasting supervisor.

CHAPTER THREE: THE PROTEIN MYTH

So insidious and destructive are the effects of a high protein diet, and so extensive is the research which proves as much, that it is difficult to understand why the 'lots of protein is good for you' myth still survives (though I think the Meat and Livestock Commission have a lot to do with it). Excess protein is so damningly implicated in premature ageing that it is hard to understand how anyone who is serious about caring for themselves in the long-term can continue to eat large quantities of high-protein foods.

A diet which supplies more protein than the body needs actually causes deficiencies of many essential vitamins, including the B vitamins, B6 and niacin. It also causes important minerals such as calcium, iron, zinc, phosphorus and magnesium to leach out of the body and, during protein breakdown, complex by-products are formed some of which are highly toxic (ammonia for example). These toxic residues deposit themselves throughout the body, predisposing it to degenerative illnesses - to arthritis, atherosclerosis, heart disease, cancer, even to schizophrenia. Lots of protein certainly brings about early and rapid growth, but it also brings about early and rapid ageing and disease[2].

One of the most dangerous protein by-products is a fatty-waxy deposit called amyloid, found in large quantities in the tissues of dedicated over-eaters of meat. Dr P. Schwartz, professor of physiological pathology at Frankfurt University and a world expert on amyloid deposits and their implications, refers to amyloid as the most important and perhaps decisive cause of decline with age. It not only stifles proper cell metabolism by interfering with the movement of oxygen and nutrients, but also damages cell membranes and DNA[1].

An excess of protein, particularly of animal origin, has been linked to a myriad of degenerative conditions, resulting in visible changes which we call ageing and in a shortened lifespan. Three German physicians called Wendt studied the role of excess protein in the diet.

With the aid of electron microscopy, they were able to show that excess protein clogs the basement membrane, which is a filter between small blood vessels (capillaries) and cells. When this filter is clean and clear, nutrients and oxygen pass through quickly and efficiently from the blood into the cells, where they are needed. Similarly, waste products of cell metabolism pass out of the cell quickly and do not poison the interior of the cell. However, the more protein your diet contains, especially protein of animal origin, the less efficient this process becomes, due to the clogging of the filter; the basement membrane. This, of course, is the beginning of degeneration, of sluggish cell functioning and auto-intoxification of cells. If this process continues for long enough, the clogging becomes so bad that insoluble protein begins to line the capillary and arterial walls, leading to arteriosclerosis, high blood pressure and adult diabetes. The cells just aren't getting the nutrients and oxygen they need. It's hardly surprising that many people feel so tired so much of the time! However, by avoiding all protein of animal origin and by eating an increasing amount of foods in their raw state you may be able to reverse this process. As previously mentioned, raw vegetable protein is easily assimilated and does not lead to this clogging of the basement membrane. On a totally raw food regime, and once the body is sufficiently detoxified, nutrients and oxygen can go straight through into the cells. The basement membrane should become thin and porous again[3].

As Carl Pfeiffer, author of 'Total Nutrition', says 'There is a general belief that only meat gives us protein and that vegetables could never be equal. This is quite erroneous. It is a matter of calorie density: for instance, a helping of broccoli has a very high protein value in proportion to the calories consumed. There is also the advantage that the calories are in a high fibre form (cited in [1]).

An over-consumption of protein has been linked to breast, liver and bladder cancer and to an increase in the incidence of leukaemia[4]. Uric acid is one of the most potent poisons known and high-protein foods, especially flesh foods, are a major source of uric acid. When autopsied, all victims of leukaemia show a high uric acid level in their blood *which would decrease on a low-protein diet.* Uric acid is responsible for both gout, an extremely painful and deforming type of arthritis, and uric acid kidney stones. Both are prevented _and_ healed with a low-protein diet. Calcium kidney stones, very painful and the most common type of kidney stone, is also the result of a high-protein diet. They too can be prevented by lowering animal product consumption.

As already indicated, protein is the most difficult food for the human body to deal with and because of the strain imposed by processing excessive protein, the liver and kidneys are over-worked and they enlarge. It has been shown that people experiencing kidney or liver failure improve dramatically when a low protein diet is taken[4].

Because of propaganda, fuelled by commercial interests, we consume far more protein than our body's require. The RDA (Recommended Daily Allowance) is set at 55 grams per day. However, it has been shown that we only need about 30 grams or less per day, but the World Health Organisation (WHO) nearly double that figure to add a 'margin of safety' (on average, most people in the West are taking in about 100 grams a day)([4]).

Unfortunately, the idea that we need so much protein is based on tests conducted on animals (rats). However, I think it is plainly obvious WE ARE NOT RATS!! We are led to believe that animal products are the best source of protein, when it has been demonstrated over and over again that a diet totally devoid of animal products can supply us with all the nutrients that our bodies ever need. On the other hand, the excess protein which our body's can't use, for instance, on an animal-based diet, is broken down into amino acids, some of which are metabolised in the liver and excreted into the urine, together with large amounts of minerals. One of these minerals commonly lost is calcium! **Studies show that the more protein you consume, the more calcium you lose!! (Ibid.).** This was demonstrated as far back as in 1930, showing that, in humans, a diet with a high meat content caused the loss of large amounts of calcium, and a negative calcium balance. As an example, Eskimos consume one of the highest protein diets in the world, and they also have one of the highest incidences of osteoporosis in the world. They are already stooped over in their mid-twenties. In fact, where protein consumption is highest, osteoporosis is most common (Ibid.).

As you are probably aware, the craze of a high-protein diet has been sweeping across America, Britain and the rest of Europe over the past several years, both as a slimming diet and a diet 'prescribed' for diabetic patients. This diet can be fatal and will not promote slimming or diabetes control in the long-run, in fact, on the contrary - it will only lead to further ill-health.

It is a fact that most people in this country are slowly, and some cases quickly, dying from malnutrition - that's poor nutrition. They overfeed on high-protein foods at the expense of carbohydrate foods and this, in turn, leads to heart disease, cancer, diabetes, kidney disease, osteoporosis, etc., etc. I repeat, most people in the Western world have an excess of protein (and fatty) foods, usually in the form of animal proteins.

These high-protein, low carbohydrate plans differ in details but they share some common claims([5]):

Myth 1: If we eat too many carbohydrates, we'll have too much insulin in our bodies. Excess insulin places us in what one writer describes as 'carbohydrate hell'. The result is supposedly an increased risk of heart disease, cancer, arthritis, and a host of other health problems.

Myth 2: Human beings originally enjoyed a diet that was high in protein. Our bodies are genetically-adapted to this way of eating.

Myth 3: You can lose weight quickly and permanently by consuming more protein and eating fewer carbohydrates.

These diets therefore advocate a high animal-protein diet, rich in all flesh foods, eggs and milk, etc., but low in carbohydrate foods like fruits and vegetables.

The Facts
High-protein foods are likely to be high in cholesterol and saturated fats - substances that can promote heart disease and various cancers. Weight loss from high-protein diets comes at first from losing water. However, long-term weight control means losing fat, a goal that calls for changing eating habits

over time and from taking more exercise. On high protein diets people can temporarily lose large amounts of weight, and can even lower their blood cholesterol, sugar, and triglycerides, says John McDougall, M.D. (cited in [5]), but the method is unhealthy. On a very low-carbohydrate diet, like the Atkins diet, the body burns fat, and the by-products of this are ketones, which suppress the appetite and can cause nausea. Dr McDougall points out this same condition of ketosis occurs when people are ill; so they are freed to rest and recuperate, rather then be forced by hunger to gather and prepare food - because they simulate a state seen with serious illness.

These diets contain significant amounts of the very foods, i.e. meats, that the American and British cancer societies and heart associations tell us contribute to our most common causes of death and disability. The reason blood cholesterol, sugar, and triglycerides may be reduced on high protein diets is that people are eating much less because of their loss of appetite, and sometimes nausea. In general benefits are temporary because it is too unpleasant to be sick - so people go back to their old way of eating!

I, of course, would agree that you can manipulate symptoms through diet, but I would qualify that manipulation is not the same as healing and furthermore, it does not address the cause of the problem. Protein has such a high profile - courtesy of the meat and dairy industries.

A while after certain people eat carbohydrate foods they experience sudden drops in their blood sugar and they may experience symptoms such as lethargy and fatigue, poor concentration, mood swings, "foggy" brain, misperceptions, panic attacks, hot and cold sweats, and heart palpitations. The cause of this could be an inappropriate insulin response - too much insulin being secreted bringing the blood sugar levels down too much. However, when these sufferers are recommended by some doctors and scientists to adopt high protein/low carbohydrate diets their symptoms abate, according to Kathryn Alexander of the Gerson Institute([6]), because protein doesn't stimulate such a strong insulin release as carbohydrate. However, she argues that continuing the high-protein diet is what caused the diabetes or blood-sugar imbalance in the first place, and continuing will not make us any healthier, in fact, quite the contrary!

Recently there has been a new wave of what's called "hyper-insulinaemia", where we have moved on from hypo-glycaemia (low blood sugar) to high amounts of insulin in the blood stream. Alexander argues that the symptoms appear to be more-or-less the same, along with the discovery of excess insulin in the blood stream. What's the answer? Well some doctors argue that they need to reduce the secretion of insulin by omitting carbohydrates and increasing your protein intake. However, as soon as you go back on the carbohydrates the symptoms return. Not only this - six months down the track on such a diet you start to experience new symptoms of a more chronic nature. Excess protein creates acidity and puts a strain on the kidneys which will later affect the heart as well as other areas of the body, as previously mentioned.

Good quality protein is, of course, essential for growth and tissue maintenance particularly during infancy, childhood, adolescence and pregnancy. The growth spurts from childhood through to adolescence are controlled by high levels of growth hormone and the sudden increase in sex hormones which, during puberty, rise to eight times the adult levels. Growth hormone and the sex hormones begin to fall after puberty until they reflect the stable adult levels by the early 20's.

High protein intake on its own will not increase muscle size. Muscles store a very limited supply of protein and after this capacity is reached, excess dietary protein has to be broken down and discarded. Exercising increases muscle tone and size because the more you work your muscles the greater their capacity to store carbohydrate fuel (not protein - muscles do not use protein for energy). Beware of the high protein message if you are seeking fitness.

In order for the body to heal, no matter what the imbalance, it has to release its toxic load and rebuild its nutrient status. When this occurs, the vitality rises and healing begins. The body's intelligence will determine which areas will be healed and in what order. So again we see that the answer to disease lies in a plant-based diet, not in a calorie-rich but nutrient-devoid animal-based one.

SECTION TWO

FLESH FOODS & THEIR RELATIONSHIP TO HUMAN DISEASES

INTRODUCTION

The following chapters will make reference to the main types of animals which are farmed for their flesh and which, as a consequence, humans regularly eat. Let it be noted, however, that the restriction to these particular animals only as regards to distressing and dangerous diseases does not indicate that it is only these animals that have such diseases, nor does it mean that those diseases mentioned are an exhaustive list. For instance, ducks and other animals that people regularly consume are, of course, also subject to similar diseases on an increasing scale.

However, due to the lack of available research and papers printed on the subjects (due to obvious reasons!), this discussion will be narrowed down to a few main headings.

CHAPTER FOUR: THE DANGERS OF EATING SHEEP AND LAMBS

Even though sheep and lambs are reared less intensively than most other farm animals, they are still subject to a wide array of diseases, mostly caused by neglect rather than as a direct result of being pushed to their productive limits as cows, pigs and hens often are. However, production diseases are becoming more common in Britain's flocks, as sheep rearing becomes increasingly intensive.

Mad Sheep Disease

According to a recent report in the New York Times([3]), U.S. Agriculture officials state that a herd of Vermont sheep are suspected of being infected with a form of "mad cow" disease and have been shipped to an Iowa laboratory where they'll be slaughtered and tested. Federal agents wearing bullet-proof vests swooped down on a sleepy Vermont farm and seized a flock of sheep possibly infected with a type of deadly "mad cow" disease. The extraordinary move was the first of its kind in the United States, which until now had all but escaped the mass hysteria sweeping Europe.

The flock is one of two that had been quarantined in Vermont since 1998, after four of the animals showed signs of transmissible spongiform encephalopathy, or TSE, according to the USDA. TSE is a class of neurological diseases that includes mad-cow disease (bovine spongiform encephalopathy, or BSE) and scrapie, a sheep disease that poses no threat to humans(?). While there has never been a reported case of a sheep contracting BSE outside the lab, the USDA says it doesn't want to take a chance. The always-fatal human form of BSE is contracted by eating contaminated beef. "It's possible for sheep to contract the cattle version of the disease. We don't know," said Jim Rogers, a USDA spokesman in Vermont.

The government says the sheep may have contracted mad-cow disease or a new species of scrapie after eating contaminated feed before they were imported to the U.S. from Belgium in 1996. The animals have been used for breeding and for milk for fancy cheese, some of which has been served in upscale New York City eateries. There is no known transmission of either disease through milk, the scientists say.

Other Diseases

According to Penman([1]), the drive for multiple births is increasing the level of lamb and ewe mortality. Pregnancy toxaemia or twin lamb disease caused by the uterus pressing on the ewe's digestive system, can restrict her food intake which weakens the ewe and her lambs, and reduces her output of sufficiently high quality milk. Poor quality milk leaves the lambs open to a range of opportunistic diseases, including a bacterial infection known as watery mouth or rattle belly. This is generally diagnosed by a 'splashing sound if the lamb is gently shaken'. Other symptoms are a distended stomach and incessant drooling.

Many sheep suffer from foot rot which often results in lameness (what of lamb chops you may be asking yourself). The increasing use of high-density housing and pens is believed to be contributing to this problem.

Sheep scab is also a major problem. It is combatted, together with blow-flies, by sheep dipping, using organophosphate pesticides (Ibid.). These pesticides are a possible cause of BSE. These compounds, which were discovered during the search for battlefield nerve gasses, killed virtually everything in the animal's wool and on its skin and are highly toxic both to the farmer and the sheep. In October 1994, the *Sheep Farmer* warned shepherds that 'uncontrolled nervous signs' can result from using the wrong concentration, or even if the farmer or his animals should swallow some of the agent. The symptoms of organosphosphate poisoning include 'excessive salivation and tears, frequent urination, vomiting, difficulty in breathing, muscle twitching developing to uncoordination, paralysis, collapse and death. In 1985, twice yearly sheep-dipping was made compulsory to try to stamp out sheep scab and blow-flies but, following concern about the health effects on the farmer, it was made optional again in 1992. In addition, users of the sheep-dipping compounds must now obtain a competence certificate before they may do so.

Sheep may also contract scrapie, from which BSE is supposed to have originated (the contributing factors are controversial). The symptoms include teeth grinding and lip twitching. If the animals are startled they may fall into an epileptic fit. They suffer from intense itching and lose all co-ordination. Paralysis is swiftly followed by death. There are no reliable estimates of the incidences of scrapie in Britain because it is not a notifiable disease. As The British Veterinary Association said in a memorandum to the House of Commons: "We can only guess at the incidence of disease. There has been an omission." (cited in [1]).

Most animals with scrapie, which has an incubation period of 18 months-5 years, are eaten (before the first symptoms appear) and have been for many years with no *known* ill-effects, so despite its link to BSE, scrapie is thought to be unlikely to spread to humans(!)(Ibid.).

Pushing animals to their biological limits is not only an issue for people who care about animals, it is of concern to anyone who cares about their own health and well-being. Mad Cow Disease, Salmonella, Listeria, chicken cancer, etc. have all shown what happens when humanity tampers with the food supply. With BSE, the human victims may only run into thousands, but it may also reach epidemic proportions.

In recent years, some of the government's top advisers on mad cow disease have stopped eating British lamb for fear that it might contain the deadly nvCJD prion. A full-scale search has been launched to see if sheep have contracted the diseases and if they have, it is rumoured that the entire British flock of 20 million animals will be slaughtered. Professor John Collinge, a member of the government's BSE team, warned that there could be risks from lamb, contaminated blood products and surgical instruments[2]. Further, according to the January-March 2001 issue of 'The Food Magazine' there is evidence that sheep may carry the cattle disease BSE according to very recent studies.

CHAPTER FIVE:
THE DANGERS OF EATING PIG MEAT

Since February 2001 the media has bombarded the British publish with scenes of devastation across the country. Foot and Mouth disease amongst pigs, sheep and cows has spread like wildfire causing many farm animals across Britain to become infected. And the answer? Kill all known infected animals and those in infected areas as a precautionary measure. Soldiers have been brought in to accommodate MAFF's (the Ministry of Agriculture Fisheries and Foods) demands and aid in the massacre of thousands upon thousands of animals, even ones in labour. The British Government's relentless attack on these animals has turned many, many people vegetarian almost overnight. The cost to the environment of the dioxin exposure from the funeral pyres is yet to be seen in full force, but the weather changes in England are the first obvious signs.

Meanwhile, it appears that the British government's motives are purely economic. Foot and Mouth is not a serious disease amongst livestock in general, except for the very young animals, and as such only results in flu-type conditions. Even humans who it is claimed have caught Foot and Mouth in the human form have reported on only flu-like symptoms. Amongst the allegations, rumour has it that this is a desperate attempt to declare Britain a disease-free country as far as live exports are concerned. Whatever the motive behind these events, it is clear that vegetarianism is now, more than ever, very much on the increase.

Diseases In General
Despite the use of drugs and disinfectants, intensification of pig production have, in recent years, created disease problems including viral pneumonia, meningitis, swine vesicular disease, blue-ear disease and scours (diarrhoea). To reduce their losses, farmers resort constantly to doping the pigs with drug cocktails to manage the ever-present threat of an epidemic killing or weakening their stock and reducing the profit margins. Due to the 'factory farming' of animals including pigs and piglets, bone and joint diseases are also at

59

epidemic proportions amongst them because the animals are forced to grow faster than their bodies can cope with([1]).

In August 2000, there was news of a severe outbreak of swine flu, of which we are told by newspapers, 'cannot spread to humans' (Daily Mail 19.08.00). However, *just to be cautious*, many thousands of pigs were prematurely slaughtered. Isn't it amazing how the government are erring on the side of caution when it is obvious to all thinking people that sick animals will inevitably lead to ill-health in humans when they are consumed.

In an article by the PCRM, by Neal D. Barnard, M.D. and A.R. Hogan([2]) state that when you bite into a hot dog you're asking for trouble! If a standard ten-pack of hot dogs observed the truth in labelling, here's how its ingredient list might read: Carcasses from old or thin cattle and swine; cheeks, jaws, hearts, tongues, lips, eyelids, gums, intestines, ears, nostrils, tails, snouts, tendons, windpipes, livers, kidneys, salt, fat, bones, blood and preservatives.

In fact, laboratory tests conducted in 1993 by the Los Angeles Times found that one-fifth of the major-brand hot dogs analysed contained a bacterium called Listeria monocytogenes, which often triggers flu-like symptoms and, in some cases, even more serious sicknesses. In March, Ball Park Brands hot dogs were recalled from fifteen states in America (Ibid.). Three other studies, published in June 1994 in the medical journal 'Cancer Causes and Control', indicted hot dogs and especially their preservatives called nitrites as possibly cancer-causing. Girls and boys who ate a dozen or more hot dogs monthly developed childhood leukaemia at nine times the usual rate. Expectant mothers who ate at least one frankfurter weekly doubled their child's risk of getting brain tumours. Likewise, with the daughters and sons of fathers who ate hot dogs before their conception. A typical hot dog has a dozen times the fat content of a bowl of oat bran, is also high in sodium and cholesterol and contains not one speck of fibre, unless it comes from rat droppings(!). If grilled, the cooking process can produce carcinogenic heterocyclic amines on the hot dogs' surfaces. Hot dogs also pose a fatal choking hazard, especially for children under age five (Ibid.).

60

As Suzanne Havala, R.D., author of the American Dietetic Association's 1993 vegetarian position paper, put it, "The nutritional merits of regular hot dogs are few and the demerits are many." Of course, hot dogs constitute only a small facet of the health-negating, meat-and-dairy-centered standard Western diet (cited in Ibid.).

Neal D. Barnard, M.D. and Karen Pirozzi[3] say that the same pig who melts your heart on the big screen will contribute to clogging it up if you eat him for dinner. Everyone needs to consider the health consequences of consuming Babe's relatives, or any other animal. Regardless of what pork producers would have us believe, the other white meat is anything but health food. It's disheartening to hear people think they're doing themselves a favour by switching from red to white, from burgers to chops, or to drumsticks or fillets. Barnard and Pirozzi argue that, in fact meat and other animal products contain dangerously high levels of fat and cholesterol, the leading causes of heart attacks, strokes, many cancers, and a battery of other chronic and life-threatening diseases. The American Dietetic Association acknowledged the healthfulness of the vegetarian diet in a 1997 position paper and more physicians, who on the whole received an abysmal amount of nutrition training, are beginning now to join the ranks of such renowned doctors as Dean Ornish, John McDougall, and the late Benjamin Spock, all avid advocates of adopting a vegetarian diet.

More than seventy percent of the 119 million U.S. pigs expected to be killed for food in 1998 lived out their short lives in grossly over-crowded factory farms. Such conditions lead to diseases for which the animals repeatedly receive antibiotic treatments. Traces of those drugs get passed along to consumers, most of whom are as oblivious to that danger as they are unaware of the pigs pitiful lives (Ibid.).

To worsen matters from a health perspective, economic imperatives increasingly pressure farmers to produce heavier pigs who fetch heftier prices, hence the addition of growth-stimulants to the genetically-manipulated pigs' antibiotic-laden diet. Because that pound of pork you eat today in his or her former life consumed pounds and pounds of grain, you also get lots of pesticides - as much

61

as 14 times the pesticides found on even conventionally-grown vegetables (Ibid.).

Pig AIDS

More recent research has highlighted yet another disease affecting pigs, according to ABC News in a report entitled 'AIDS-Like Symptoms Threaten Pigs'. They say that a disease in pigs, similar to human AIDS, appears to have hit some pigs in the United States. The reporter, Nicholas Regush argues that this horrendous disease, which has been called swine mystery disease, blue abortion, and swine infertility, is now referred to as Porcine Reproductive and Respiratory Syndrome, or PRRS. This disease has infected some pigs in about 75 percent of American pig herds according to experts. Vaccines have only partially been effective. The disease also has been creating a nightmare for many other nations since at least the mid-1980s. The reproductive and respiratory syndrome, which often kills baby pigs, is characterised by a variety of conditions and is causing economic hardship for pig farmers. Affected mothers lose up to 10 percent of their pregnancies. Their babies are spontaneously aborted or are stillborn. As many as 20-30 percent of survivors may suffer and die from respiratory disease, such as pneumonia.

The PRRS virus is said to primarily attack a pig's immune system, leaving the body open to a host of other infections, particularly in the lungs. Some pigs develop a chronic infection and become carriers but show no symptoms. Research reveals that the virus is transmitted via semen, saliva and blood. Those pigs herded closely together and transported at close quarters by trucks may be more susceptible to infection. However, to date, there is no confirmed evidence that the virus can infect humans from any source, including via food.

Scott Dee with the University of Minnesota College of Veterinary medicine, a PRRS researcher, says the disease is the most economically devastating swine disease there is, and that the problem is getting bigger. Furthermore, Monte McCaw, a PRRS researcher with North Carolina State University's College of Veterinary Medicine, believes that while the differences between PRRS and AIDS are obvious to researchers, it is also important to study the similarities.

<u>Some Similarities to AIDS</u>
McCaw has concluded that the following key conditions in PRRS-infected pigs are similar to what is found in AIDS:

Secondary infections, mainly in the lungs, are common due to the immune-suppressive abilities of the PRRS virus.

PRRS reproduces in cells called macrophages, which are front-line cells in the body's immune system.

PRRS primarily reproduces in cells called alveolar macrophages, which are immune cells in the lung. Damaging these lung immune cells makes the animal susceptible to opportunistic infections.

Key white blood cells of the immune system (lymphocytes) go through some of the same changes that occur in AIDS.

Lymphocytes produce higher levels of a variety of biochemical substances, as in AIDS.

McCaw adds, however, that the baby pigs that manage to survive the onslaught of infections in the lungs that the PRRS virus triggers end up thriving. This is an obvious difference in the way (AIDS and PRRS) generally develop, he says.

A recent finding shows PRRS can be transmitted from one pig to another via the repetitive use of (vaccination) needles, Dee argues. He also says that PRRS hides out in the lymph nodes. The same is claimed for HIV. There may well be a number of factors that initially combine to trigger PRRS. The disease has often been referred to as a mystery, and in many ways it remains so. While progress has been made, no-one should be over-confident about any aspect of this terrible disease in pigs.

CHAPTER SIX: FISH AND SEAFOOD - THE _UN_HEALTHY OPTION

Examining Some of the Myths about Fish

Some people think that fish lead free lives before they are caught but, increasingly, more and more fish are reared under artificial conditions. For instance, in salmon farms fish are confined in underwater cages (breeding grounds for disease and parasites) and fed a diet of pellets impregnated with dyes to colour their flesh pink. One of these dyes canthaxanthin is banned in the U.S.A. and Japan, because it is a known cancer-causing agent.

There is also the mistaken belief that fish don't feel pain, however, all animals need the ability to feel pain in order to survive, and to help them to escape danger, or to encourage immobility of a wounded part of the body as an aid to healing. Fish possess a nervous system and do feel pain. Fish often die slowly without being slaughtered from asphyxiation; they literally drown out of water as we would drown in water. In fish farms, they are hauled in from the sea in their wriggling thousands and left to suffocate or to freeze to death when they are packed in ice. Some fish, like trout for instance, are caught by a line and fight furiously for their lives with a hook impaled through their sensitive lips.

Around 30,000 tonnes of farmed salmon are slaughtered each year in Britain. After a period of starvation (of up to two weeks), salmon are hit on their heads or placed in a tank with carbon dioxide bubbling through, or sometimes with an electric current before being bled to death. At sea, dynamite is sometimes used to render the fish unconscious in a particular area and the edible ones are selected. Poisons such as cyanide may replace the dynamite, in which all fish and corals are killed, whether edible or not.

On fish farms, pesticides are used regularly, the most toxic of which is Aquaguard, which is used to control sea lice. The active ingredient in Aquaguard is one of the most poisonous to be found on the Department of the Environment's dangerous substances red list[2].

65

The Fish Oils Scam

Although fish and fish oils are often touted as health promoters, they certainly are not when you consider the facts. Fish oils are extracted from the liver of fish. Just as with the liver of humans, a fish's liver is the central organ for processing chemicals, so accumulations of toxins in the fish such as mercury and other heavy metals, PCB's, radioactive material, DDT, dioxin, sewage, antibiotics, oestrogens, etc., mainly concentrate in the liver. Do you really want to be consuming this?

The idea that fish oils are healthy and that they protect arteries is based on the notion that Eskimos do not suffer heart disease or strokes, but what is seldom mentioned though is that they decrease the blood's ability to coagulate and stop bleeding! Eskimos are said to be free from heart disease due to the huge amount of fish they eat, but did you know that they suffer from the world's highest rate of cerebral haemorrhagic strokes, nosebleeds and epilepsy? Simply put, the fish oil that reduces platelet stickiness and clotting and the incidence of heart attacks in Eskimos is also responsible for their commonest cause of death: cerebrovascular haemmorhage; their blood taking up to an hour to clot. They also have the highest rate of osteoporosis in the world[3].

The Cholesterol Connection

Fish eating also contributes to gall bladder disease and **the flesh of most fish is high in cholesterol** (as mentioned, cholesterol concentrates in the lean part of animal flesh). According to Dr Neal Barnard[6], many people believe that fish is good for the heart but fish are definitely not a healthy food to consume. He quotes in his article a study published by 'The New England Journal of Medicine' which that those who followed a diet emphasising poultry and fish found that their cholesterol levels changed very little. The reason for this is that fish flesh contains plenty of cholesterol and fat, just like beef! Fish also contains approximately 15-30% saturated fat, which is lower than the saturated fat of beef and chicken, but still much higher than truly low-fat vegetarian foods. In fact, Dr Barnard argues that the only diet which actually reverses arterial blockages is a low-fat vegetarian diet.

66

Dean Ornish, M.D., carried out a study of patients suffering from heart disease and compared patients on the chicken and fish diet recommended by the American Heart Association (AHA) as against those following a strict vegetarian diet only including small amounts of skimmed milk as an optional extra. The majority of those following the AHA guidelines got progressively worse, while those who made intensive changes to their diet got progressively better.

Omega-3 Fatty Acids

Regarding the much-touted Omega-3 fatty aids, Dr Barnard argues that although omega-3 fatty acids can normally reduce the level of triglycerides in the blood which plays a role in heart disease, those that are found in fish are highly unstable. The fatty acids found in fish have the tendency to decompose and unleash dangerous free radicals, which are linked to cancer, arteriosclerosis and premature ageing. According to researchers at the University of Arizona (Ibid.), the omega-3 fatty acids found in vegetables, fruit and beans are more stable than those in fish, in addition to being coupled with antioxidants, which can help to neutralise free radicals. Fish can also contribute to cancer in other ways, argues Dr Barnard. They carry contaminants from polluted waters and about 40% of fish samples have so much bacterial contamination that they have already begun to spoil before they are sold (Ibid.). Therefore, fish, far from being brain food may actually inhibit the brain and the nerves thanks to the mercury content.

Dioxins from Eating Fish

Recently, the British Dietetic Association have advised people not to eat more than one piece of oily fish a week because of high levels of poisonous chemicals (obviously they would not advise people to stop eating fish entirely, due to financial interests). Dioxins and PCB's have been detected in all fish, but are particularly high in mackerel, herring and other species where oil is distributed throughout the animal's flesh. They can cause cancer, are thought to have a 'gender bending' effect and can cause birth defects ([5 & 6]). Consumer Reports found PCB's in 43% of salmon, 50% of whitefish and 25% of swordfish([6]).

According to the New York Times([8]) in a recent report, fish oil and fish meal have the highest level of dioxins out of all foods. Dioxins, which are produced as a waste product by industrial plants and waste incineration, have been linked to hormone changes, cancer in animals and other severe disorders. Scientists have called for changes in the levels of dioxin considered acceptable for human consumption. "Nobody is saying we can't eat fish anymore, but consumers must be made aware that fish contributes significantly to the intake of dioxins," said Johan Reyniers, a European Union spokesman. This is particularly true, he said, for fish from the more polluted areas like the North Sea (where much of British fish comes from) and the Baltic around Scandinavia.

The warning about fish comes as Europeans are already panicking about the spread of mad cow disease and the consumption of beef is dropping drastically. Dioxins were included in the global ban that was negotiated recently by representatives from 122 nations, but specialists said it would take time for countries to carry out the provisions of the treaty, which is to be signed in May 2001. The ban will affect dioxins and a dozen other toxic, long-lasting chemicals - "persistent organic pollutants" - that are recognised as a threat to the environment, and to human health in particular.

According to the new report, fish meal and fish oils of European origin have dioxin levels up to eight times as high as similar products from non-industrial regions. The fish meal and fish oil also contain up to 10 times more dioxins than are found in meat and eggs. **This is troubling because the fish meal is used in the diets of farmed fish and other food animals like chickens and pigs.** Dioxins are also found at higher levels in carnivorous fish like salmon, eel and trout than in herbivorous ones the scientists said. The new report by the Scientific Committee on Food, and a second one by the Committee on Animal Nutrition, are not binding on the European Union countries, but their opinions are generally treated seriously. The studies were made at the request of the European Union after a scare last year, when Belgian animal feed was found to be laced with dioxins as a result of a factory mix-up.

Responding to complaints that food safety standards are too lax all over

Europe, the European Union ordered a wide study of dioxin contamination of food and feed. If stricter limits for dioxins are set, related legislation is expected to provoke opposition from the strong fishery lobbies in North European countries, which have a sizeable fish-meal industry. Europe produces 500,000 tons of fish meal a year.

Dangerous Levels of Mercury Found in Fish

As if the dioxin and cholesterol problem with fish isn't enough, another recent report, published by CNN entitled 'Fish-Mercury Risk Under-Estimated'[9] tells us that millions of pregnant women and their foetuses are at risk of serious health problems from exposure to mercury in fish. Of course, as a general rule, what is not safe for mothers and babies is also not safe for the public at large. The report, prepared by the Environmental Working Group and the U.S. Public Interest Research Group, calls on the Food and Drug Administration to upgrade and strengthen its current mercury safeguards. The new report, "Brain Food: What Women Should Know About Mercury Contamination in Fish," contends the recommendations do not go far enough to protect women and children from mercury contamination. In addition, the report says canned tuna, mahi-mahi, cod and pollack should not be eaten more than once a month. The widespread contamination of fish with mercury has given its reputation as 'brain food' a new and disturbing connotation," said Environmental Working Group analyst Jane Houlihan, principal author of the report. "Mercury is toxic to the developing foetal brain, and exposure in the womb can cause learning deficiencies and delay mental development in children."

Under the FDA's current recommendations, pregnant women can safely eat up to 12 ounces per week of cooked fish not on the risk list, but Richard Wiles - the Environmental Working Group's senior vice president - said that even this amount could cause problems. "Hundreds of thousands of women would get unsafe exposures to mercury if they followed the FDA's advice and ate freely of all fish in the food supply except the four that they've prohibited during pregnancy," Wiles said. Mercury contamination is equal to lead contamination as a public health issue affecting children. "It's a major public health failing on (the FDA's) part," Wiles said, "and we feel quite strongly that they need to aggressively look into the problem of mercury contamination of fish, expand the list of fish that women need to avoid and get this information out to the medical community and to women in a much more aggressive way." The biggest source of mercury pollution in our environment is coal-fired power plants. Once in the environment, mercury enters waterways and accumulates in the muscle tissue of fish. Fish and other seafood products are the main source of methylmercury toxicity in humans, and foetuses are particularly vulnerable. The report is based on the examination of 53,000 records of mercury test results in fish from seven federal, state and other government sources in the U.S.

A 'KIRO-7 Eyewitness News Consumer Reporter reported in June 2001([10]) that there's new evidence claiming that there's enough mercury in canned tuna to cause concern.up until now no-one has ever told pregnant women to totally stay away from tuna, however, recent studies suggest that even a tiny little amount of mercury can harm a developing human brain. Consumer Reporter tested dozens of cans and pouches of tuna recently and researchers claim that they found reason for concern.

According to Consumer Reporter: "Considering the the large amount of canned tuna that's eaten, we found levels of mercury high enough to pose a risk to a vulnerable group." The question here is that if tuna fish might harm a developing brain, what can and will it do to an already-developed one? Mercury has an affinity for the pituitary gland as well as other body organs and can clog up our bodies and lead to all sorts of diseased states.

Other Problems with Fish

A recent newspaper report also tells us that shellfish contaminated with a poison-causing Amnesic Shellfish Poison (ASP), which has been the cause of death for 20 people in Canada, have been found off Scotland's west coast, and more than 8,000 square miles of fishing grounds, home to the 'finest' scallops, have been put off limits, according to a recent newspaper report. The contamination is blamed on ammonia effluent - four times the permitted EU level - from Scottish salmon farms which, say environmentalists, feeds naturally-occurring algae which produce the toxins. The estimated discharge of ammonia from West Coast salmon farms into Scottish waters equals that from the raw sewage produced by over 7 million people (The Mail on Sunday 18.7.99).

In Britain, in another recent study, this time by The Ministry of Agriculture, Fisheries and Food found dioxins and PCB's - two of the World's most dangerous poisons - in *all* samples of different brands of fish fingers available in supermarkets. Both chemicals are linked with cancer and can cut sperm counts, reduce fertility and lead to genital malformation. (Metro 20.9.99).

Dr Barnard and Cindy S. Spitzer of the PCRM state that more than 100,000 Americans become sick through the consumption of contaminated seafood each year and that, despite tests that may be carried out, one cannot tell whether the fish one buys at a store is loaded with disease-causing bacteria, mercury, or anything else. Such traces are invisible, and government inspectors will not routinely use the sophisticated tests that could reveal the contaminants. Meanwhile, the seafood safety issue is ignored and the reality is that eating sea animals - even freshly killed, cleanly handled sea animals - can endanger one's health. The widely held public perception of seafood as health food is simply very false. The flesh of fish and other sea animals comes loaded with highly toxic chemical residues, which bioconcentrate in their muscles (the parts generally served). Fish and shellfish also contain too much protein, fat, and cholesterol to be a healthy option[7].

Of course there are lots of fish who swim the global ocean, picking up toxic pollution from places you would never dream of having lunch. **Big fish eat little fish, and the bigger the fish (such as tuna and salmon), the greater the bio-accumulation of toxic chemicals throughout their flesh.** Fish and shellfish contain toxic chemicals at concentrations as high as nine million times those found in the polluted water in which they swim. Mercury, something especially high in tuna and swordfish, can cause brain damage. Pesticides, such as DDT, PCBs, and dioxin, have been linked to cancers, nervous system disorders, foetal damage and many other health problems. **Avoiding fish eliminates half of all mercury exposure,** and reduces one's intake of other toxins as well (Ibid.). Of course, avoiding all animal products avoids a large majority (up to 90%) of all pesticides and herbicide residues, etc.

Also, evidence shows that women who often eat fish are more likely to give birth to sluggish infants with small head circumferences and learning disabilities than women who rarely or never eat fish. In fact, nursing infants consume half of their mother's load of dioxins, PCBs, DDT and other deadly organochlorides (Ibid.).

Contrary to the myths, fish are a relatively high-fat food and up to 30% of their fat is saturated fat. Fish such as salmon and trout have a high-fat content and accumulate hormone-disruptors and persistent organic pollutants (POPs). Canadian scientists suspect that any fish that migrates between fresh and salt water may be especially vulnerable to high concentrations of environmental eostrogens because these fish must undergo major hormonal changes to adapt to salt water. On the other hand, top-predator fish are likely to be the mot contaminated with mercury, a heavy metal hormone disruptor and shellfish tend to concentrate cadmium, another hormone disrupting heavy metals ([11]).

Of course, as mentioned, even eating fresh, relatively pollution-free fish (if you can find them) does not promote good health as fish flesh provides excessive amounts of protein, fat and cholesterol, with no fibre, complex carbohydrates, or vitamin C. The consumption of animal protein often increases bone calcium loss, encouraging osteoporosis ([7]).

Nowadays, many people eat fish rather than beef in the hope of limiting fat and cholesterol, however, many fish including catfish, swordfish, and sea trout contain almost one-third fat (saturated fat also contributes to degenerative disease). **In fact, salmon is fifty-two percent fat and ounce for ounce, shrimps have double the cholesterol of beef.** The Physicians Committee for Responsible Medicine argue that fish and fish-oil capsules contain an unhealthy amount of artery-clogging saturated fat and that studies show that diets based on fish do nothing to reverse arterial blockages. Moreover, **blockages continue to worsen for patients who regularly eat fish.** Fortunately, eating vegetables such as broccoli, lettuce and beans provides essential fatty acids in a more stable form, with zero cholesterol and little saturated fat - a much healthier substitute! (Ibid.)

72

Therefore, mounting evidence shows that eating fish and other sea animals is extremely unhealthy. No increased vigilance to reduce the slimy bacteria on their decomposing and pollution-laden bodies will improve their inherently inadequate nutritional levels or reduce the toxic chemicals laced throughout their flesh (Ibid.). If toxic chemicals and saturated fat are not enough for fish flesh, consider that fish and the bacteria living in them flourish in cold water; often at the same temperature range as your refrigerator. Even properly handled, constantly refrigerated dead fish rapidly rot. At least forty percent have begun to spoil before being taken from the seafood counter. Any fish that smells 'fishy' is indeed spoiling. But do not rely on your nose to protect you! As much as ten percent of raw shellfish, while appearing perfectly fresh, are infected with organisms that can cause hepatitis, salmonella poisoning, cholera, and even death (Ibid.). Just how fresh do you want your saturated fat, cholesterol and mercury anyway?

CHAPTER SEVEN: WHAT EVERYONE SHOULD KNOW ABOUT POULTRY MEAT

Ian Coghill, Vice Chairman of the Environmental Health Office's Food Safety Committee says that chicken should carry a government health warning on the packet, like cigarettes.[7]

Contrary to the myths that chicken and turkey (and fish) contain less cholesterol and that, reportedly, chicken and turkey represent a good option for those on a healthier diet, Dean Ornish, M.D., reported that on a five-year follow-up of patients on his popular plan for reversing heart disease with a totally vegetarian diet, compared with patients on the chicken and fish diet recommended by the American Heart Association (AHA), the majority following the AHA guidelines got progressively worse, whilst those who made intensive changes got progressively better[4].

Plant foods contain no cholesterol but animal products always do. For every one percent increase in cholesterol levels, heart attack risks rises by two percent. For every 100 milligrams of cholesterol in the daily diet; the typical amount in a four-ounce serving of either beef or chicken, one's cholesterol level typically zooms up five points. (Unlike fat, cholesterol concentrates in 'lean meat') (Ibid.).

CHICKENS AND CANCER

Broiler hens are the chickens which are routinely used for large portions or whole portions of chicken meat. Tony Moore of Joice and Hill broiler breeders was quoted as saying that chicken cancer (Marek's disease) is responsible for the excessively high losses of chickens and, despite chickens being vaccinated against it as day old chicks, mortality is increasingly significant (cited in [1]). There is also a rapidly increasing threat from Gumboro disease, another viral cancer and, on top of this, avian leukosis a bird variety of leukaemia is now commonplace.

'Spent' battery hens are commonly found in soups, pies, etc., however, scientists have discovered that a very high percentage of battery hens develop malignant tumours of the oviduct. The

75

incidence of these cancers has coincided dramatically with the increased egg production achieved by poultry breeders over the last few decades[8]. It is therefore not surprising to learn of the recent findings suggesting that eating cooked chicken meat causes cancer.

Marek's disease is not transmitted through the egg, but commercial flocks are usually infected at an early age, passing cancer from bird to bird, often via feather follicle cells which are the most important source of infection. The acute form of Marek's disease has an incubation period of 3-4 weeks to several months. Since birds may be slaughtered before clinical signs of the disease is visible, there is undoubtedly a serious risk to all consumers of chicken and chicken products [1].

SALMONELLA
In food processing plants where they work with red meat as well as chicken, the chicken preparation areas are often cordoned off from the rest of the plant. The work there is carried out behind glass screens in a kind of quarantine just in case bugs which thrive on and in chicken leap out and infect everything else. One of the most widespread of these bugs is salmonella. Almost every process of chicken production helps to spread bugs from one chicken to another until they finish up inside the plastic wrappers. There is a danger when touching raw chicken that people can spread the infection elsewhere.

Often the inedible parts (blood, offal and feathers) are recycled to be included in the feed of subsequent batches of chickens. Salmonella bacteria are able to live in hen's internal organs for months, being excreted intermittently in droppings. If ovaries become infected, the transmission of salmonellae can be through the yolk. Many farmers selling free-range eggs buy their birds from the same breeders who supply battery farmers - the birds may be infected even before they start their egg producing life.

Once slaughtered and processed, raw chickens are frequently contaminated with dangerous pathogens. The 1987 Public Health Laboratory service figures for contamination were as follows: Salmonella 60%, Listeria 60%, Campylobacter 50%. A large

76

proportion of ready-cooked chickens on supermarket shelves have been found to harbour dangerous levels of listeria bacteria. Listeriosis can cause miscarriages and stillbirths and kills 30% of its victims (Ibid.).

MAD CHICKEN DISEASE
Startling evidence that mad cow disease might have spread to poultry is now being examined by government scientists an investigation by newspapers revealed. Ministers were stressing that they were taking seriously evidence which could spark a new crisis for the meat industry. The Ministry of Agriculture have been examining the brains of dead hens suspected of having CJD or bovine spongiform encepatholpathy (BSE) and plan to bring in an independent scientist for a second opinion. The specimens were sent to the Ministry by a BSE specialist Dr Harash Narang. This followed Jack Cunningham's decision to extend full mad cow disease controls for sheep and block imports of European beef not subject to them (Ibid.).

OTHER DISEASES AND HEALTH IMPLICATIONS
The US government allow the sale of chickens with airsacculitis, a pneumonia-like disease that causes pus-laden mucus to collect in the lungs. In order to meet federal standards, the chest cavities are cleaned out by a suction gun, but during this process the air sacs burst and pus seeps into the meat[2].

Chicken pieces are often parts of diseased hens which could not be sold as whole chickens. Approximately 36 million chickens a year die from heart attacks, fatty livers and kidneys, colisepticaemia, viral arthritis, perosis, etc. (The statistics for the different types of chicken cancer are unfortunately not available). Chickens that may be severely diseased, but not dead may be slaughtered and go unnoticed and sold in supermarkets or butcher shops[1].

Broiler sheds are never cleaned out during the lifetime of any one batch of birds, so the litter becomes impregnated with faeces. Used broiler chicken litter is fed to cattle. A series of botulism was reported in 1988 and many animals died as a result of being fed infected litter. It was reported that there were dangers of botulism being passed to humans and it is still a potential health risk to animals and humans. In the squalor of the broiler house infections spread like wildfire. Salmonella, listeria, campylobacter and botulism all thrive in the sheds and can infect the living and processed birds and form a vicious circle of disease. A huge percentage of birds processed for human consumption have these diseases. Chickens, of course, may be fed the flesh and by-products of any other animals including sheep (which may be infected with scrapie) and cattle (which may be infected with BSE), dead (through disease) chickens and chicken excrement (Ibid.).

In a very recent report entitled 'UK Watchdog Says Shop Chickens Rife with Food Bug' Britain's food watchdog said that about one in two chickens in UK supermarkets were infected with the most common form of food poisoning bacteria. The Food Standards Agency said campylobacter, which can cause severe stomach pains and diarrhoea, had been found in frozen, fresh, domestic and imported chickens across the country, with higher rates in Scotland and Northern Ireland.A survey, carried out between April and June, found 46% of chickens tested in England were infected with the bacteria, 42% in Wales, 75% in Scotland and 77% in Northern Ireland. Earlier the British Broadcasting Corporation said it had conducted a survey and had found that campylobacter was present in 69% of 100 chickens tested from Britain's leading supermarkets( ).

According to an article by Murry Cohen, M.D. and Allison Lee Solin of the PCRM([3]), Campylobacter, the most common cause of diarrhoea in the United States, can sometimes lead to a paralysis-inducing disease called Gullian-Barré Syndrome, and Salmonella which causes severe food poisoning, can be fatal. They state that, according to 1997 tests conducted by the Minnesota Health Department, seventy-nine percent of chickens sampled from supermarkets were infected with campylobacter, and twenty percent of those were infected with an antibiotic-resistant strain. About fifty-eight percent of turkeys were infected, and eighty-four percent of those carried the resistant strain. With the introduction of quinolones for use in poultry, resistant strains of campylobacter are now appearing in the U.S., explains Stuart Levy, M.D., a physician with the Tufts School of Medicine, who described the antibiotic-resistance trend as an international public health nightmare. In February 1999, the British medical journal 'The Lancet' reported that scientists had discovered antibiotic-resistant bacteria in feed being given to chickens in the United States. The authors called it an ominous sign for humans.

In the Spring/Summer 2000 issue of the Physician's Committee for Responsible Medicine newsletter([5]), Kieswer reports that chickens have been involved in a grand marketing campaign to promote them as some sort of 'health food', and with nine billion chickens eaten each year in the U.S. alone, it appears that many people have fallen for it. However, an honest look at the nutritional value of chicken reveals quite a different picture. She argues that chicken meat is not low in fat, and "not even close." A 3.5-ounce piece of broiled lean steak is fifty-six percent fat as a percentage of calories, and chicken contains nearly the same at fifty-one percent. Compare that with the fat in a baked potato (one percent), steamed cauliflower (six percent) and baked beans (four percent) and any ideas that chicken is a health food go out the window. Fancy packages can't disguise the fact that chicken and all meats are muscles, and muscles are made of protein and fat.

Kieswer further states that too much protein also puts a strain on the kidneys, forcing them to expel extra nitrogen in the urine, increasing the risk for kidney disease. Also, the combination of fat, protein and carcinogens found in cooked chicken creates troubling risks for colon cancer. Chicken not only gives you a load of fat you don't want, it's Heterocyclic Amines (HCAs) are potent carcinogens produced from creatine, amino acids and sugars in poultry and other meats during cooking. These same chemicals are found in tobacco smoke and are fifteen times more concentrated in grilled chicken than beef. HCAs may be one of the reasons that meat-eaters have much higher colon cancer rates; about three hundred percent higher compared to vegetarians.

Kieswer argues that with live salmonella bacteria growing inside one in every three packages of chicken, it is making a lot of people sick. Although deaths from salmonella poisonings sometimes make the evening news, millions more cases that cause flu-like symptoms go unaccounted. Salmonella poisoning can cause vomiting, diarrhoea, abdominal pain and low-grade fever, lasting for several days. When it spreads to the blood and other organs, it can be fatal (and is for as many as 9,000 people every year). Also, campylobacter infects as many as two-thirds of all pre-packaged chicken. Salmonella and campylobacter have become increasingly common because modern factory farms crowd thousands of chickens into tightly confined spaces, where excrement and other forms of bacteria spread contaminants. As we have learned, chicken has the same amount of cholesterol as beef; four ounces of beef and four ounces of chicken both contain about 100 milligrams of cholesterol and the cholesterol from chicken similarly clogs arteries and causes heart disease (Ibid.). The human body produces cholesterol on its own and never needs outside sources. Each added dose contributes to artery blockages which lead to heart attacks, strokes and other serious health problems.

According to Dr Barnard of the PCRM[6], chicken may look harmless but fancy marketing campaigns cannot disguise its shortcomings. Chicken may be lighter in colour than beef, but your body can hardly tell the difference. Chicken, like other animal products, contains hefty doses of cholesterol, fat, and animal protein. It leaves your body wanting for fibre, vitamin C, and complex carbohydrates. When heated, chicken produces dangerous heterocyclic amines (HCAs) as creatine, amino acids, and sugar in chicken muscles interact. HCAs, the same carcinogens found in tobacco smoke, are 15 times more concentrated in grilled chicken than beef. The fat, animal protein, and carcinogens in cooked chicken creates risks for colon cancer. What's more, poultry, like all meat, lacks any fibre to help cleanse the digestive tract of excess hormones and cholesterol. Moreover, you wouldn't dream of taking veterinary medicines, but in choosing chicken you're doing just that. Today's farms increasingly operate much like factories. Unlike PCBs, which are slow to leave our bodies, chemicals from medicated feed and various veterinary compounds do get eliminated when we stop eating meat. In comparison with the general population, vegetarian women have 98 to 99% lower levels of several pesticides as well as many other chemicals ingested by eating animal products.

In fact, a recent article in The Times reported that the growth-promoting drugs zincbacitracin or virginiamycin and antibiotics such as penicillin which are banned from chicken production in the EU to prevent the development of resistant bacteria, are freely available in Thailand and Brazil. The British food industry sources say that chicken imported cheaply from these countries is entering the country unchecked and is most likely to be used in products such as soup, pies, curries and ready meals (The Times 18.10.99).

And what about the way in which the chemicals alter and mimic our own body chemicals? In a frightening book entitled 'Hormone Deception' by D. Lindsey Berkson, the author argues that with up to 80,000 birds packed into one warehouse and fed commercial feed which contains numerous potential hormone-disrupting toxins (pesticides, herbicides, antibiotics and drugs to combat disease so prevalent when so many animals are housed together) and the rendered fat in commercial feed contributing to other toxins, chicken hardly seems like a healthy option. The ingestion of these types of chemicals may show up as disorders and cancers of the reproductive system, etc.[10]

Suffice to say, the dangers posed by eating poultry meat are therefore all too real and the poultry industry's greed has turned the bird's suffering into many, many diseases for which humans will now pay the consequences.

CHAPTER EIGHT: CAN ANIMAL CANCERS SPREAD TO HUMANS?

According to Cox in 'The New Why You Don't Eat Meat'([1]), it has taken a long time for much of the scientific community to accept that cancers could be caused and transmitted by a virus. In experiments as far back as 1911, it was demonstrated that tumours taken from one chicken and implanted into another would infect the second chicken with a cancerous growth. In 1936, it was demonstrated that breast cancer could be transmitted between mice via a virus present in milk of lactating mice. More recently, scientists at the University of Glasgow discovered feline leukaemia in cats. Today cancer-causing viruses (oncoviruses) are now scientifically categorised as a part of the retrovirus family. Despite this, the belief still partially persists that cancer somehow 'ought not' to be capable of being virally induced.

However, just like human beings, the animals we eat suffer from various forms of cancer, sometimes caused by a virus. For example:

* Bovine leukaemia virus (BLV) causes cancer of the lymph tissue in cows.

* The avian leukosis virus (ALV) causes leukaemia in chickens.

* Marek's disease virus (MDV) causes a cancer of the lymph and nervous systems in chickens.

In fact, one American report found that: virtually all commercial chickens are heavily infected with leukosis virus (Ibid.). Since the tumours induced are not grossly apparent until about 20 weeks of age, the virus is not economically as important as is the Marek's disease virus which induces tumours by 6-8 weeks of age. Bovine Leukaemia virus, however, is widespread in commercial dairy herds. More than 20% of dairy cows and 60% of herds surveyed in the USA are infected.

Now the key question is whether eating diseased meat, or being exposed to diseased 'food' animals or their produce, result in a greater likelihood of contracting leukaemia or any other form of cancer? To investigate whether these viruses can cross the species barrier and infect humans, a study was established, paid for by the US National Cancer Institute. The scientists conducting this study reported that "The viruses are widely distributed naturally in their respective hosts and are present not only in diseased, but also in 'healthy' cattle and chickens destined for human consumption" For instance, a 1972 USDA report lists carcasses passed as fit for human consumption after diseased parts were removed, which listed nearly 100,000 cows with cancer and over 3.5 million with abscessed liver (Ibid.).

Cox says that it therefore seemed logical to examine the health of those people who would have maximum exposure to these animals - slaughtermen. Accordingly, the health of 13,844 members of a meat-cutters union was checked from the period of 1949 to 1980. After statistical analysis, it was found that **abattoir workers were nearly three times more likely to die from Hodgkins disease (a cancer of the lymphatic system) than the general population.** The scientists concluded:

"The excess risk was observed only in abattoir workers and seems to be associated with the slaughter of cattle, pigs and sheep. Thus, the excess risk seems to be in keeping with a postulate of an infectious origin for these cases, as no other occupational exposure could adequately explain this occurrence".

By itself, this report is very significant. But now consider the following additional evidence:

"It has been shown in laboratory experiments that bovine leukaemia virus can survive and replicate even when placed in a human cell culture."

Indeed, scientists have found a close similarity between bovine leukaemia virus and HTLV-1 - the first human retrovirus ever shown to cause cancer.

A study recently conducted in France has concluded that the children of fathers who work in the meat trade are at greater risk of developing childhood cancer. The study examined over 200 cases of leukaemia diagnosed in the Lyons area, and found that a significantly larger number of fathers of children with leukaemia than expected worked as butchers or in slaughterhouses. The scientists suggest that the bovine leukaemia virus could be to blame (Ibid.).

Statistical analyses of human deaths from leukaemia and other cancers have shown that those people who have the most contact with 'food' animals (vets, farmers, butchers, etc.) run a significantly higher risk of dying from certain types of cancer than would be expected. For example, in a Nebraskan study, it was shown that men having regular contact with cattle were twice as likely to die from leukaemia (Ibid.).

In a study from Poland it has been shown that farmers, butchers and tanners are more likely to develop leukaemia than other people. And a further Polish study concluded:

"It should be inferred that cattle with leukaemia may, in favouring circumstances, be a factor disposing man to neoplasms (cancer), especially to the proliferation of the lymphatic system, either through longer contact with sick animals or the longer ingestion of milk and milk products from cows with leukaemia. The fact that with a rise in the incidence of leukaemia in cattle there also appears an increase in proliferating diseases in the lymphatic system is particularly worthy of attention."[1]

Cox also reports that a study conducted in Minnesota amongst leukaemia sufferers showed that a higher than expected number of them were farmers having regular contact with animals. A similar study conducted in Iowa found a relationship between leukaemia in humans, cattle density, and the presence of bovine leukaemia virus in cows.

A study of mortality from leukaemia and Hodgkins disease amongst vets has shown that they run a significantly higher risk of dying from lymphoid cancer than the norm. The vets were in clinical practice, in close contact with food-producing animals, and the authors of the report suggested that a viral cause may be responsible.

A study conducted in France and Switzerland in 1990 reveals that male breast cancer sufferers (generally rare in men), were most likely to work as butchers.

Like the French study previously mentioned, an Italian study conducted by scientists at the University of Turin has confirmed that the children of butchers are more likely to contract cancer (Ibid.). This though could be attributed to a high meat consumption, rather than to a virus.

Cox maintains that all this evidence should be considered very seriously because it has extraordinarily profound implications. Dr Viro Hube, a physician who spent 15 years as a milk inspector for the state of California, writes:

"The Food and Drug Administration states that many unanswered questions remain about BLV, such as transmission, infectiousness and whether it's a threat to humans. Some of the questions fuelling the controversy are whether the process of pasteurisation, which inhibits infection, destroys the aspect of the virus capable of producing cancer. Also, how great is the risk of pasteurised milk being accidentally contaminated with raw milk. If we wipe out BLV, will we see a reduction of those cancers related to fat consumption? In fact, might it be the viruses and not the fat that are linked to some human cancers?

Cox[3] argues that there are several possible ways in which an animal cancer virus can induce disease in humans. One theory suggests that a 'helper virus' can form an association with another relatively harmless

86

one and, in the process, produce a virus that can induce cancer. An animal virus may not, therefore, directly precipitate the disease in humans, but it may be able to convert otherwise harmless human viruses into killers.

At the moment, it has not been fully and finally proven. This is because it is ethically unacceptable for scientists to try and induce cancers in human populations for experimental purposes (though it is deemed as acceptable to induce cancers into animals). Nevertheless, the circumstantial evidence is strong enough to allow us to ask the question whether we can get cancer from eating cancerous meat.

However, in some ways the connection is really very simple. Firstly, we know that some 'meat producing animals' (especially cows and chickens) suffer from tumours and cancers. Secondly, we know that cancer can be transmitted by virus, from one animal to another and indeed from one species to another. Thirdly, cancerous and tumourous meat are not necessarily removed at the slaughterhouse, and may quite easily find its way to the butcher's shop.

The inevitable conclusion drawn from the above is that the chances are that if you eat meat, sooner or later you will eat part of an animal that either has cancer or has been exposed to a virus that can cause cancer. It is difficult, however, to quantify the risk you would be running by eating tumourous meat (especially since cancers can take many years to surface).

Here is a summary of the evidence currently available that supports the cancer and meat connection (Ibid.):

- It has gradually been proven that a considerable number of viruses can be passed from animals to humans - some examples being rabies, yellow fever, cow pox and encephalitis (BSE). Additionally, some viruses may only produce cancer in humans, not other animals, and be very slow acting.

- Marek's disease (a scourge amongst chickens) is caused by a Herpes virus. A recent scientific report established that 'there is a strong association between the possession of antibodies to Herpes simplex virus (HSV) type 2 and cervical carcinoma of women.'

- One study has shown that a 'helper virus' can form an association with another relatively harmless one and, in the process, produce a virus that can induce cancer. One such virus (the Rous sarcoma virus) occurs in chickens. **There is, therefore, a possibility that such a virus may enter the human body and convert harmless human viruses into killers.**

- In one experiment, humans already suffering from advanced cancer were inoculated with a virus that was known to cause cancer amongst monkeys. The patients all developed the same tumours as the monkeys. A laboratory worker also inoculated himself by accident, and developed a tumour.

- Cows, chickens and turkeys are known to suffer from leukosis, a form of cancer that is known to be produced by a virus. Leukosis produces multiple tumours, and sometimes goes on to produce leukaemia in the animals too. **It has been shown that virus-like particles exist in the milk taken from herds of cows where there is a high incidence of leukosis.**

- It has been shown in experiments that Bovine Leukaemia Virus (the virus that causes leukosis in cows) can survive and replicate itself when placed in a human culture.

- Another report investigated an outbreak of leukosis amongst cows in a dairy farm in the United States, and found that over a ten year period two farm employees and two farm neighbours all developed leukaemia of the same type.

- Extensive experimental work with the viruses that cause leukosis in poultry has proven that they can be transmitted from chickens to other animals, including rats, mice, hamsters, guinea pigs, rabbits, frogs and monkeys and, (more to the point!) it has also been shown that these viruses can infect human cells kept in experimental cultures.

So what does all this add up to? It suggests that at least some of the meat eaten today comes from animals that are suffering from some form of cancer, which can possibly infect humans.

Of course, meat is supposed to be inspected at the slaughterhouse, however, Cox asked one veterinary surgeon with responsibility for meat inspection to tell him what regulations, if any, applied to tumourous carcasses. He was told that meat hygiene regulations were difficult to enforce, particularly with regard to poultry. "It's the feeling of many Official Veterinary Surgeons that poultry inspection standards are being whittled away," he told him. "Until we joined the EEC, the inspection was pretty minimal in any case. Nevertheless, the standards are dropping again. For example, if you're someone who rears and kills your own birds (and many people do), then there's no requirement for any inspection at all". "What about tumours and other cancers in meat?" Cox then asked him. He pulled out his file concerning the Meat Inspection Regulations and said "It's an interesting situation". "If a carcass contains just one tumour, then it would be cut out of the carcass and condemned, but the rest of the carcass would be passed."

"So no-one would ever know that the animal had cancer?" Cox then enquired. "That's right" he said. "But if the carcass contains two or more tumours, then the whole carcass would be condemned. It could then go for pet food." Although sometimes condemned meat has a habit of turning up as fit for human consumption. Cox then said "I understand that a meat inspector on a poultry line has three to five seconds to examine each bird and judge whether it's healthy". "Is that sufficient time to give it a clean bill of health, free from tumours?" The vet smiled and told Cox that, even with his experience, he couldn't perform an autopsy that quickly.

In this chapter we have examined some crucial issues regarding animal and human disease connections, and the relationships between meat consumption and the occurrence of certain forms of cancer. Cox argues that it will certainly be many years before every feature of the complex process of zoonotic carcinogenesis has been resolved and that there will, no doubt, be many people who will not wish to see these rather dark and disquieting fringes of medical and veterinary knowledge examined too closely....

CHAPTER NINE: HEALTH RISKS RELATED TO BEEF AND VEAL

In the past decade or so stories have cropped up in the media about the possibility of BSE spreading to people, however, these were generally dismissed as scares by the Government and the meat industry repeatedly said that the public had no need to be alarmed! They talked about the safety of British beef, instead of ways of eradicating the disease, and castigated the media for whipping up 'scare stories'.

In 1990 a BSE-type disease took hold in a herd of kudu at London Zoo. At about the same time, gemsbok and nyala, who were thought to have eaten scrapie-infected meat both succumbed to a spongiform disease at Marwell Zoo, as did a cheetah who is believed to have eaten cattle meat that contained infected spinal material

The Medical Research Council decided to investigate, and conducted a trial involving four marmoset monkeys to see if BSE could infect primates. Two were injected with material taken from scrapie-infected sheep, the others with tissue taken from BSE-infected cows. In December 1991 they announced the results. The two marmosets that were injected with material from scrapie-infected sheep died of a spongiform disease but the two injected with material taken from BSE-infected cows appeared alive and well. 'Beef given clean bill of health' said the headline in the Meat Trades Journal !([1]). A few months later, however, the headline changed: 'Primates are affected by BSE'. This followed a Medical Research Council announcement that the marmosets injected with material taken from BSE-afflicted cows had died of a spongiform disease.

Was this the nail in the coffin for British beef? Not quite. The experiment had one flaw: It had been designed to see whether BSE could take root in primates. It could never be proven that it can be transmittable under normal circumstances *between* other animals or species. So the nagging doubt remained. Could it infect humans? MAFF continued trying not to answer the question in any meaningful sense. In November 1992, after a series of feeding tests on cuts of beef, they concluded that there was no risk to humans (Ibid.).

However, several independent scientists did not believe the reassurances! Dr Steven Dealler, a consultant micro-biologist, says that 75% of animal species exposed to the BSE causing agent developed the disease. Therefore, he concluded that humans have a strong chance of susceptibility to it. His work, which he admits contains a high degree of uncertainty, concludes that **if it spreads to humans, the disease could kill anywhere between 10,000 and 10 million people.** The reason for this wide margin is that we currently know little about spongiform diseases. Estimates vary, but as little as one teaspoon of infected cattle feed may in time be enough to kill a cow. Nobody knows for certain whether this amount, or in fact any quantity, is lethal to humans.

The BSE Crises
Dr Dealler and other scientists who suggested that BSE may spread to humans were widely regarded as lunatics until 20th March 1996 when Stephen Dorrell, the Secretary of State for Health at the time, was forced to admit for the first time that BSE may spread to humans and cause Creutzfeldt-Jacob Disease.

CJD is usually rare in humans, about one case per million people per year and is constant throughout much of the world. It is also predominantly a disease of the elderly. But scientists working for the National CJD Surveillance Unit noted that in 1994 the disease pattern had changed; it was beginning to occur in younger people and, by the end of 1995, ten cases had been reported. Not many, perhaps but at the start of an epidemic there are only ever a handful of sufferers.

Dr Rob Will, Head of the National CJD Surveillance Unit said: "We are reporting a new phenomenon, a major cause for concern". Professor John Pattison of The Spongiform Encephalopathy Advisory Committee (SEAC) announced that "We have now arising in 1994 and 1995, ten cases of a varient of CJD that we have not seen before. The incubation period of spongiform encephalpathies is five to fifteen years. This suggests that something new happened in the middle of

92

1995 that would have resulted from exposure in the middle to late 1980's. This drives us inevitably to the conclusion that the most likely risk factor for these cases in the middle of the 1980's is exposure to BSE" (Ibid.).

The Government was forced to admit that its previous attempts to contain BSE had failed, and new guidelines stipulated that all cattle over thirty months old from BSE-infected herds and about 100,000 others thought to be most at risk of the disease were to be slaughtered, rendered and incinerated at the end of the 'useful' lives. It also tightened the rules on rendering and meat and bone-meal (believed to have caused BSE and which was finally banned from the animal food chain). All animal feed that may have contained rendered animal waste was to be recalled, and its possession became a criminal offence.

Could these measures have worked? According to Steven Dealler, they will remove the majority of infected material from the human food chain but will do little to eradicate the disease. It is possible that, if these measures had been adopted when the disease originally appeared, that by now BSE would have been long forgotten, and there would have been no threat to the public health - but that, of course, would have affected the profits of the meat industry. The Government and the meat industry, of course, preferred to keep the money coming in!

Naturally, BSE seems to be spreading from cow to calf, which means that the disease is endemic to the dairy herd, but there have, as yet, been no studies showing that it may spread through cows' milk. Meanwhile, MAFF clings to the belief that cows are still becoming infected through contaminated feed, which shows that renderers and slaughtermen are still failing to obey the law and guard the health of consumers and farm animals. If the disease is endemic, as appears likely, then the only solution to the meat industry is to destroy all infected herds (Ibid.). (Of course, a more simple and better solution would be for humans to stop eating animal flesh!).

The majority of the infected material was officially removed from the *human* food supply in the late 1980s but still some leaked into cheap meat products such as burgers and meat pies. Therefore, an unknown number of people may have already taken a lethal dose of the BSE-causing agent. A slow disease may already be chewing its way through their nervous system, and there is nothing they can do about it. Whether they ate the disease-causing agent as a result of government incompetence in delaying the removal of infected material from the human food supply, or the meat industry greed in flouting the rules and allowing the material to 'leak' into the food chain is another question.

One recent indication, however, from a recent report in the Daily Mail states that, according to researchers, deaths from the human form of mad cow's disease are rising by about a third every year. It is feared that the increase could signal the start of an epidemic caused by BSE-infected meat products. In the first six months of the year 2000, fourteen Britons died from vCJD - the same amount as those who died last year. A further six people are suspected of having the fatal brain disease. The analysis by the National CJD Surveillance Unit in Edinburgh published was published in the Lancet on 4th August 2000. It shows that deaths have increased every year since 1995 when the first seven cases were recorded. By June 2000, seventy-five cases in total had been reported including sixty-nine deaths. Dr H. Ward, one of the investigators, said that the figures are 'a cause for concern'. Furthermore, Simon Cousens from the London School of Hygiene and Tropical Medicine who helped produce the report said that it is the first time that we have clear evidence that the figures are increasing. Some experts fear that as many as 500,000 Britons could die over the next thirty years.

In May 2001, it was reported by BBC News that one hundred people have now died from the human version of mad cow disease v-CJD. Government scientists warned that the number of cases could be gathering pace. However, some scientists had predicted that the number of fatalities would never reach three figures. Last year the total number of confirmed and probable cases was 28. So far this year (5 months into the year) the figure has reached 16. Professor Roy Anderson from Imperial College, London, a member of the

Spongiform Encephalopathy Advisory Committee (SEAC) said: "Last year was bad news, and this year looks as if it's going to be higher than last year. "It will be a long time before we have an idea of the scale of the epidemic. "The bottom line is that the future is still uncertain. "All I can say at the moment is that I doubt that it's going to get better."(2)

BSE, has since been reported in other European countries and suspected in the United States. It has also been reported more recently that sheep and lambs have a version of mad cow disease too. BSE-type symptoms have also arisen in other farm animals including chickens and pigs.

Veal and Calves
Many people are already aware of the cruelty inflicted on the veal calves, as there has to-date been much publicity directed towards highlighting the attrocities of the veal crate system. However, many people do not realise that aside from the obvious cruelty, the calves are fed on canned powdered milk complete with antibiotics and hormones (to increase growth rate and prevent disease) and eventually all manner of processed foods including newspaper, animal testes, gristle, entrails and parts even unfit for putting into hamburgers. Their saturated fat levels are high since they are confined to in crates and do not graze or freely exercise. Any animal fed in this way often develops cancer very early on and a lot of it does not get removed during butchering(3).

Therefore, cows and calves, do not seem like a healthy option in the light of the aforesaid. In this chapter, we have examined how government inefficiency and greed has allowed the escalation of a crisis that might have long ago been contained. Humans are now becoming victims of yet another disease to add to the list of diseases of which they were already suffering from. Although the cause of the BSE crisis still remains quite controversial, there nevertheless seems to be a connection between eating infected animals and vCJD.

SECTION THREE

DIETARY-INDUCED HUMAN DISEASES

INTRODUCTION

Animal flesh and animal products have been known as contributing factors in the cause of many human diseases. Among the most prominent wastes that a human being can load his body with are urea and uric acid (nitrogen compounds), which are found in the body following meat consumption). For example, beefsteak contains fourteen grams of uric acid per pound of meat. This means that the kidneys of meat-eaters are worked three times more in the elimination of poisonous nitrogen compounds in meat than those of vegetarians. The reason for this is that although carnivores have the enzyme uricase to break down uric acid, humans who are frugivores by physiology, do not. When kidneys can no longer handle the excessively heavy load of a meat diet, the unexcreted uric acid is deposited throughout the body. It is absorbed by the muscles like a sponge soaking up water, and later it can harden and form crystals. When this happens in the joints, the painful conditions of gout, arthritis and rheumatism result; when the uric acid collects in the nerves, neuritis and sciatica result. Now many doctors are now advising patients who suffer from these diseases to stop eating meat([1]).

Uric acid is one of the most potent poisons known and high-protein foods, especially flesh foods, are a major source of uric acid. When autopsied, all victims of leukaemia show a high uric acid level in their blood. Uric acid is responsible for both gout, an extremely painful and deforming type of arthritis, and uric acid kidney stones. Both are prevented and healed with a low-protein diet.

Calcium kidney stones, very painful and the most common type of kidney stone, is also the result of a high-protein diet. They too can be prevented by lowering animal product consumption. Protein is the most difficult food for the human body to process, especially in its cooked state, and because of the strain imposed by the processing of excessive protein, the liver and kidneys are over-worked and they enlarge. It has been shown that people experiencing kidney or liver failure improve dramatically when a low protein diet is taken ([1]).

Also, since our digestive system was not designed for a meat diet, poor elimination is a natural consequence and is a distressingly common complaint of meat eaters. Meat, being extremely low in fibre, has this major disadvantage - it moves very sluggishly through the human digestive tract (4 times slower than grain and vegetable foods) making chronic constipation a common ailment in our society. Much recent research has shown conclusively that a healthy elimination pattern requires the bulk and fibre available only from a proper vegetarian diet. According to present research, natural fibre may be a significant deterrent of appendicitis, diverticulitis, cancer of the colon, heart disease and obesity[1].

The above, therefore, gives us some insight into some of the reasons why meat is harmful, as well as the many other reasons which the reader has now learned of. Let us now proceed to address some of the most notorious complaints which are mainly suffered by those adhering to a meat-based diet.

CHAPTER TEN: ARTHRITIS AND RHEUMATISM

Arthritis is a specific term describing inflammation of the joints. Rheumatism is used more broadly and describes all aches and pains in the muscles, bones or joints. In this sense, we have all suffered from rheumatism at some time. Rheumatoid arthritis is inflammation and pain of the joints and the surrounding tissues.

Many different causes have been suggested for these diseases, including stress, allergies, food and environmental pollution, malnutrition, hormonal imbalance and digestive inadequacy[1]. Conventionally, however, the medical profession have treated the idea that arthritis may be diet-related as unsubstantiated folklore. As recently as 1990, for example, the University of California's own health publication advised its readers that "no dietary regimen or nutritional supplement has been shown to alleviate or prevent arthritis"[1]. Nevertheless, the evidence has been very forthcoming!

According to Cox (Ibid.), meat and dairy foods contain arachidonic acid, and it has been demonstrated that levels of this in the blood fluctuate according to the consumption of these products and can indeed promote joint inflammation. He argues that adopting a vegan diet can significantly reduce arachidonic acid and the subsequent pain of arthritis, as the following studies prove:

- In one study of rheumatoid arthritis, published in 1986, patients were asked to fast for a week, which was then followed by three weeks of a vegan diet. At the end of this time, 60% said they felt better, with less pain and an increased functional ability.

- Some people may be particularly sensitive to dairy products. In one experiment, a 52-year old white woman who had suffered with arthritis for eleven years was tested to see which food provoked her arthritis the most. Eating normally, she would suffer about thirty minutes of morning stiffness, with nine tender joints and three swollen joints. After a three day fast there was no morning stiffness. However, when she was given milk (the study was blinded so she didn't know what she was swallowing), the arthritis returned with a vengeance with thirty minutes of morning stiffness, fourteen tender joints and four swollen joints.

- In The Lancet in 1991, it was reported that twenty-seven patients were asked to follow a modified fast for 7-10 days (herbal teas, vegetable broths and juices were included) and they were then put on a gluten-free diet for three and a half months. The authors of the study had already accepted that fasting was beneficial, but that most patients relapsed on return to food. Gradually the subject's diet was altered by adding a new food item every other day, eventually arriving at a lacto-vegetarian diet for the remainder of the study. If the introduction of one food produced symptoms, then it would be eliminated again. A control group ate an ordinary diet throughout the whole study period, for comparison purposes. After four weeks the vegan diet group showed a significant improvement in the number of tender joints, swollen joints, pain, duration of stiffness, grip strength and many other measurements of health. The scientists reported that "the benefits in the diet group were still present after one year".

Dr Robert Gross states that he has had innumerable arthritics recover normal joint function through fasting followed by a vegetable, fruit and raw nut regime. The fast promotes detoxification of the body and a marked improvement, both in general health and in local conditions follows. Relief from excruciating pain is gained within only a few days after the fast is instituted. A marked reduction of swelling and enlargement of the joints, restoration of motion in the stiffened parts and great comfort and ease are immediately enjoyed(2).

Dr Herbert Shelton described a case where a lady with arthritis recovered completely after a fast. She was 44 years old and her arthritis was very painful and crippled her movements. Her physician could promise her nothing but temporary relief with drugs for the rest of her life. Dr Shelton fasted her for three weeks and it freed her of all pain and inflammation and restored normal movement to her joints. After the fast she remained free of all pain and inflammation of arthritis (Ibid.). Our bodies have an amazing self-healing ability when given the right conditions. When the body is freed up and can release some of its toxic load, it can do wonders! Of course, for continued success, dietary choices following the fast are of crucial importance.

CHAPTER ELEVEN: OSTEOPOROSIS

Osteoporosis literally means porous bones. Both men and women can suffer osteoporosis, but it is more common in women, according to Cox[1]. Osteoporosis is caused by a slow loss of bone mass. Eventually, the bones will become brittle and will break very easily. In some women this process is sufficiently slow to avoid fractures and pain. On the other hand, some post-menopausal women, within 10 years of the menopause, suffer such significant bone loss that they will easily fracture their hip, etc. The conventional treatment is Hormone Replacement Therapy (HRT), even though some studies show that oestrogen therapy (HRT) may *increase* the risk of cancer. Indeed, common 'side effects' are gallstones, weight gain and return of bleeding (Ibid.).

According to the Physician's Committee for Responsible Medicine (PCRM)[2], some studies have suggested that vegetarians may be at a lower risk of developing osteoporosis than non-vegetarians. Marsh (1988) found bone loss to be considerably less in post-menopausal women who were vegetarian than those who were non-vegetarian. The non-vegetarian diet contained higher amounts of sulphur, which derived from animal protein and dietary sulphur increases the acidity of urine, which results in increased urinary calcium loss. Increased urinary calcium loss is related to increased calcium loss from bone tissue. The PCRM point out that, in another study hip fractures associated with osteoporosis have been shown to be higher in countries consuming a diet high in animal protein (Abelow, 1992).

According to H. and M. Diamond[3], bone mass does not necessarily have anything to do with bone strength. For instance, fluoride causes bone mass to increase dramatically, but decreases its strength. This is why elderly populations in highly fluoridated communities show an increase in osteoporosis. Similarly, some drugs may increase bone mass by 5%, but because bone structure has been damaged, it isn't strengthened with the drug.

The Diamonds report some significant studies, including the following:

* Some researchers report that what presents as an absence of low bone density is a meaningless indicator of risk of fractures or osteoporosis. In a nine year study of a thousand middle-aged women, the group considered at high risk of osteoporosis actually had fewer fractures than the group not considered at risk. Bone density screening has never been shown to be effective in preventing fractures, according to a large review of published work on bone density screening.

* Regular weight-bearing exercise has consistently been shown to stave off bone loss, even in post-menopausal women. In fact, regular exercise has been shown to halve the risk of hip fractures[3].

* The usual drugs for osteoporosis, such as Oestrogen, Calcitonin or Etigronate (called 'anti-resorbing' drugs) eventually *stop* bone formation. Also, a British association called Group Against Steroid Prescriptions polled its 15,000 members to document how common side effects from steroids are. Among other side effects, half of the people reported they developed osteoporosis (Ibid.).

* A large-scale review of thirty-one studies on osteoporosis concluded that oestrogen did not have a 'significant benefit' in slowing the onset of osteoporosis.

* Another study found Oestrogen did not strengthen bones in women even when they had used it for 16 years! There is, indeed, evidence that HRT contributes to osteoporosis. Dr John McLaren Howard, a Medical Researcher from Biolab in London, studied the levels of nutrients necessary for bone development in women with osteoporosis, particularly the enzyme alkaline phosphotase. This enzyme works with magnesium to form calcium crystals in the bone, and so indicates whether new bone is being laid down. Dr McLaren found that the lowest levels of alkaline phosphotase

in the study were found in women with osteoporosis on HRT. Dr Melvyn Werback states that calcium intake is disturbed by the typically high phosphorous diet of the West. As calcium is needed to metabolise protein, a high protein diet means calcium is constantly leached from the bones. Osteoporosis is virtually unknown in places such as Africa, where far fewer proteins are eaten.

It is worth noting what happens when one has an excess of protein in the diet. When protein intake is in excess of our requirements, the excess is broken down into amino acids, as mentioned and, excreted into the urine with the excess protein, go large amounts of minerals! One of the minerals lost is calcium. Studies in fact show that the more protein you consume, the more calcium you lose. In 1930, the first study was published that showed that, in humans, a diet with a high meat content caused the loss of large amounts of calcium and a negative calcium balance[3]. Many people who think they have a calcium deficiency are on highly acid diets, so the calcium in their bodies is constantly being used to neutralise the acid. In fact, although milk and cheese are recommended to restore calcium levels in osteoporosis, because most milk drinkers and cheese eaters consume pasteurised, homogenised, or otherwise processed products, their calcium intake is unusable by the body. This processing degrades the calcium making it very difficult to utilise. In fact, contrary to the opinion of many, **DAIRY PRODUCTS ARE A MAJOR CAUSE OF OSTEOPOROSIS!** (Ibid.).

Also, foods which are high in phosphorous lead to calcium deficiencies (which would include meat and animal products). In actual fact, the body's need for calcium is filled a lot more easily than most people realise. Once that need is met, that's it! Adding more isn't going to help, in fact excess calcium in the body has *very* serious consequences, particularly in its inorganic (cooked form). It has been shown clearly that when calcium is lost from the bones, it is not just eliminated from the body. This calcium in the body is picked up by the blood and deposited in the soft tissues - the blood vessels, skin, eyes, joints and internal organs. This calcium combines with fats and cholesterol in the blood vessels to cause hardening of the arteries. The calcium that ends up in the skin causes wrinkles, in the joints it crystallises and forms very painful arthritic deposits, in the eyes it takes the form of cataracts and in the kidneys it forms hard deposits known as kidney stones (Ibid.).

Due to propaganda, fuelled by vested interests, we consume far more protein than our body's require, which contributes to a loss of calcium, as mentioned. The RDA (Recommended Daily Allowance) is set at fifty-five grams per day, however, it has been shown that we only need about thirty grams a day or less. As mentioned in the 'Protein Myth', Eskimos consume one of the highest protein-rich diets in the world, and they also have one of the highest incidences of osteoporosis in the world. They are already stooped over in their mid-twenties.The calcium-depleting effects of proteins are not lessened even when *large* doses of supplementary (inorganic) calcium are ingested. This is because mineral tablets and cooked calcium, which is in its inorganic form cannot be readily utilised by the human body. The body can only utilise raw calcium, namely from raw plant sources.

So what creates the problem of osteoporosis? Several influences have been identified: Tobacco, alcohol, caffeine, soft drinks, salt, antacids, insufficient exercise, lack of sunshine, acid-forming foods - but *the number one cause of osteoporosis is animal products! (Ibid.).*

So what can one do if they think they may have osteoporosis? Well, for a start, calcium is found in all foods grown in the ground. They easily supply a sufficient amount of calcium to meet the requirements of both growing children and adults. Animals consume the plants and absorb the calcium - that's where the cow gets calcium! However, calcium loss can be due to many dietary and environmental factors, so the best way forward would be to seek the advice of a Natural Hygienic practitioner (for more information contact the author).

According to the Life Science Institute in Canada[4], bone calcium is at dangerously low levels in those using meat as compared to vegetarians, especially in people over fifty. A high-protein diet (especially one of animal protein), increases the urinary excretion of calcium. Thus vegetarians are less prone to osteoporosis.

H. J. Curtis (in *'Biological Mechanism of Ageing'*) gives supporting evidence to the theory of animal protein causing osteoporosis. He argues that calcium is transferred from the hard tissues (bones) to the soft tissues (arteries, skin. joints, internal organs and eyes). As we have found, the transfer of calcium to the soft tissues results in many health problems including catastrophic fractures, hardening of the arteries, wrinkling of skin, arthritis, the formation of stones, cataracts, high blood pressure, degeneration of internal organs, loss of hearing, senility and cancer. Indeed, a study of elderly female vegetarians at Michigan State University showed them to lose less bone to osteoporosis than another group of the same age that ate meat[4]. Athletes who eat lots of meat are especially susceptible to arthrosis, a degenerative process of the joints. Among twenty conventional-diet, professional football players who were observed for eighteen years, 100% incidence of ankle arthrosis and 97.5% incidence of knee arthrosis were found[4].

Therefore a negative calcium balance can be easily produced by an increased protein supply and that the minerals potassium and magnesium, are also known to be deficient in an every day diet rich in meat, eggs, cheese and fat, however, they are richly present in a plant-based diet containing a large proportion of uncooked plant foods (Ibid.).

CHAPTER TWELVE:
MEAT, LEUKAEMIA AND CANCER

Harvey and Marilyn Diamond([1]), after researching hundreds of scientific journal articles and studies, argue that **animal products cause cancer, among which are cancer of the colon, breast, liver, kidneys, prostate, testicles, uterus and ovaries.** Also, over-consumption of protein has been linked to breast, liver and bladder cancer, and to an increase in the incidence of leukaemia.

Apart from the fact that human's are not physiologically adapted to the consumption (and, of course, the diseases that most farm animals are plagued with nowadays), this may be due to some of the chemicals given to animals destined for slaughter which are very dangerous. This can include penicillin, tetracycline, sewage-sludge pellets decontaminated with caesium-137, radioactive nuclear waste, fattening agents and a list of other chemicals and antibiotics to "prime" the animal for sale. Also, the chemical treatment which some meat receives when it is routinely dipped in sodium sulphite (to decrease the stench of decay and turn it red rather than the sickly grey colour of ageing animal flesh) is thought to be carcinogenic. In fact, even cement dust is included in farm animal's feed! 'Nutrition and Health' reported in 1981 that some cattle farms in the Mid-West were feeding their steers hundreds of pounds of cement dust to 'get their weight up' for sale. A consumer group, hearing of this ploy, asked the FDA to halt it and the FDA, after investigation, stated that since there has been no indication of harm to humans by ingesting some cement dust, the practice can continue until some harm is proven! (Ibid.).

Some examples of the types of poisons we consume when we eat flesh foods and its products include the following: Hydroperoxide, alkoxy, endoperoxides from heated meat, eggs and pasteurised milk; Ally aldehyde (acrolein), butyric acid, nitropyrene, nitrobenzene and nitrosamines from heated fats and oils and indoles, skatoles, nitropyrene, ptomatropine, ptomaines, leukomaines, ammonia, hydrogen sulphide, cadaverine, muscarine, putrecine, nervine and mercaptins in cheese([9]). It is, of course, no coincidence that since the proliferation of processed foods, beginning in about 1950, cancer rates steadily increased and are now at an all-time high.

In *The Encyclopeadia of Vegetarian Living*([2]), Cox states that a study conducted among 50,000 vegetarians (Seventh Day Adventists) revealed results that shook the world of cancer research. The study clearly showed that this group has an astonishingly low rate of cancer. All types of cancer occurred at significantly lower rates, as compared with a group matched on age and sex. **The study showed that their life expectancy is longer and that they had only a 53% risk of dying from cancer than the norm.**

Cox reports how the research came about. Apparently, when these scientists began to study facts and figures concerning cancer mortality in different countries, they found something very odd. It appeared that certain countries had a much higher mortality rate than others, and they began to wonder why the U.S., for example, had a much higher mortality from cancer than, for instance, Japan. They then tried comparing the amount of animal protein that different nations consume, and their cancer mortality, and the relationship became clear. There was a clear relationship between the amount of animal protein in a nation's diet and incidence of certain types of cancer mortality. But this was not the only connection. The same connection appeared with the total fat consumption and cancer, animal fat consumption and cancer and various other factors as well. To eliminate various other possibilities, they carried out more research. For instance, if the root of the problem was genetic, then it would not affect immigrant populations, but the place of birth did not seem to matter. This proved that environmental, not genetic factors, were involved. They then selected one group which was of particular interest, the American Seventh Day Adventist (SDA) population. They were subjected to repeated studies because they differed in their dietary regime since it appeared that they ate a completely different diet to the average American one.

As you are probably aware, the average American diet involves the consumption of a large amount of meat and animal products - in fact

112

up to seven or more times per week, whereas with the SDA group, half of them did not consume meat or animal products at all. They do not smoke or drink (although in the study one third of the men were previously smokers) and they tend to practice a healthy lifestyle that emphasises fresh fruits, whole grains, vegetables and nuts. A seven year scientific study then began in order to tabulate the death of 35,460 SDA's.

The scientists found that the death rate amongst SDA's was about half that of the general population - it was shown that they had a 53% incidence of death from cancer as when compared to the norm. Some of this could probably be attributable to abstinence from smoking – cancer of the respiratory tract, for example, is only 10% of the general population, but other cancers such as gastrointestinal and reproductive cancers are not causatively related to smoking.

Another study set out to check these remarkable findings, this time studying cancers of the large bowel, breast and prostate – the three most common non-smoking related cancers. As many as 20,000 SDAs were studied and, this time, they were compared to two other population groups. Firstly, their statistics were compared to the cancer mortality figures for all U.S. whites, then to a special group of 113,000 people who were chosen because their lifestyle closely matched the SDAs – except for their diet. In other respects, such as place of residence, income and socio-economic status, the third group very closely matched the SDAs. The results were dramatic. For all three cancers, deaths amongst SDAs were much lower than in other groups!

Another study took place in Israel revealing the connection between both fats from animal sources and fats from plant sources in connection with increased mortality rates. The study followed the Jewish population as it grew from 1.17 million in 1949 to 3.5 million in 1975, over which period meat consumption increased by 454%, and the death rate from malignant cancers doubled (Ibid.).

Another group of scientists, this time in Canada, studied the relationship between meat consumption and breast cancer. They

113

found that the rate of breast cancer increased with the consumption of pork and beef (Ibid.). In 1981, another massive statistical study of 41 countries, including the US and the UK, was completed. The results confirm the connection between eating meat and the risk of certain types of cancer. Yet again, they show that plant foods seem to confer protection (Ibid.).

In 1988 in Germany, a five year study of vegetarians was carried out in which a total of 1,904 participants were recruited. Deaths from all causes were very low indeed - only 37% of the average meat eating population. **In fact, all forms of cancer were slashed to 56% of the normal rate and heart disease was down to 20% (Ibid.).**

So why is cancer so typical on a meat-based diet? In recent years, there has been much research carried out to discover why it is that a vegetarian diet confers so much protection against cancer and other diseases. One theory is that vegetarians and vegans consume food that is rich in substances which suppress free-radical formation. Up to now, some sixty diseases have been linked to free radical activity including Alzheimer's disease, arthritis, MS and cancer. Further, as we have already found, the animals that many people consume are infected with cancer e.g. bovine leukaemia causes cancer of the lymph tissue in cows, avian leukosis causes leukaemia in chickens and Marek's disease causes cancer of the lymph and nervous system in chickens. One American report found that virtually all commercial chickens are heavily infected with leukosis (Ibid.).

Cox argues that one reason that meat-eaters get more cancer might be the fact that when animal flesh is several days old it naturally turns a sickly grey-green colour. The meat industry tries to mask this discolouration by adding nitrites, nitrates and other preservatives. These substances give the meat a red/pink appearance, but in recent years many of them have repeatedly been shown to be carcinogenic (cancer-inducing). On the other hand, another possible reason for the meat-cancer link may be the fact that chemicals such as DDT tend to accumulate in animal tissues, and may be found in animal tissues years after their usage has been controlled or stopped. According to Cox[2], some experts have pointed out that carcinogenic, fat-soluble

114

contaminants such as drugs and pesticides may be the reason why meat causes cancer.

However, whether it is the chemicals in animal protein which cause cancer or whatever, **the fact is that there is a link between eating meat and cancer** and it seems pretty clear that cutting out meat is a sensible way to cut down protein, which when consumed in excess, seems to be implicated in all manner of disease.

Dr Neal Barnard of the Physicians Committee for Responsible Medicine, in reviewing recent research findings, states that it has long been known that cooked red meat contains cancer-causing heterocyclic amines, which form as the meat is heated, but **the US National Cancer Institute have shown that oven-broiled, pan-fried or grilled/barbecued chicken carries an even bigger load of these carcinogens than does red meat. In fact, they argue that chicken is far more cancer-causing than red meat** (the number of PhIPs in a well-done steak contains about 30ng/g, but grilled chicken reached 480ng/g). These dangerous chemicals are strongly linked to colon cancer, but may also contribute to breast cancer[3]. Conversely, Dr Barnard also mentions that the cholesterol content of chicken is actually the same as that of beef, and the fat content is not much different either. Carcinogens are more concentrated in many cooked chicken products.

Therefore, the chemical poisons directly or indirectly added to flesh foods and the way in which many flesh foods are cooked promotes further problems for flesh-eaters. In fact, barbecued beef, for instance, contains an average of nine micrograms of benzopyrene, a cancer-producing agent. The fat dripping into the fire changes the chemical properties of the fat and the benzopyrene goes up in the smoke from the charcoal and coats the steaks[4].

Numerous researchers have linked protein with cancers of the breast, prostate, endometrium (the lining of the uterus), colon and rectum, pancreas and kidney. The type of protein which is most likely to cause cancer is the protein found in meat. The United States Surgeon General's Report 'Nutrition and Health' said: "In one international correlational study, for example, a positive association was observed between total protein and animal protein and breast, colon, prostate, renal and endometrial cancers (Armstrong and Doll, 1975). Similarly, a migrant study indicated an association between meat consumption and cancer of the breast and colon (Kolonel, 1987)." The Surgeon General also reported that: "Studies have also found an association between breast cancer and meat intake" (Lubin et al, 1981).

A diet primarily consisting of raw plant foods increases cell oxygenation, which is a critical factor in cancer prevention. This is just as important in the healing of a sick body as it is in protecting against illness, including cancer. In the development of most chronic illness, regardless of the specific disease, lowered cell respiration is evidenced, according to L. and S. Kenton. Nobel Laureate Otto Warburg, Director of the Max Planck Institute for Cell Physiology in Berlin, discovered for instance that while normal cells use oxygen-based reactions as their source of energy, cancer cells are different. They tend to derive their energy from a glucose-based energy instead. Other researchers, such as Heinrich Jung and P. G. Seeger, confirmed Warburg's work and showed that cancer, as with many other degenerative diseases, arises from a disturbance in cellular respiration, which results not only in a lowering of energy, but in a serious disturbance in metabolism in the organism as a whole. When normal cell respiration is restored by a raw diet, the vitality of the whole organism and its immunity to disease, is increased([7]).

Also, several studies have shown a relationship between incidence of prostate cancer and the consumption of animal protein. Because most people who eat a lot of meat usually also eat a great deal of fat (because meat often contains a lot of fat) it is difficult to know whether these links between meat and cancer are a result of the protein in the meat or the fat in the meat. (Of course, many people think that they can just cut away the fat, but the problem is that the actual flesh often still contains a lot of fat!). It is also possible that the link between meat and cancer is a result of mutagens being formed during the cooking of meat.

Some of those who advocate meat-eating claim that vegetarians are likely to have a diet that is deficient in iron. This, of course, is nonsense. A good, well-balanced plant-based diet will contain plenty of iron. Indeed, there is now evidence to suggest that too much iron in the blood (a problem which can occur among meat-eaters) increases the chances of cancer developing. When iron has been absorbed, the body stores it. In many Westernized countries, iron 'overload' is thought to be more common than iron deficiency (Ibid.). The American Physician's Committee for Responsible Medicine report that: "higher amounts of iron in the blood mean a higher cancer risk". (It also appears that iron that comes from animal sources called haem iron is more likely to cause heart disease). Diets of vegetables, legumes, fruits and grains provide adequate iron. Plant-based diets, for instance in China, typically contain more iron than is consumed in the US[4].

Cox argues that dairy product consumption has also been associated with iron-deficiency in some infants, both because dairy products are very low in iron and because they can stimulate occult intestinal blood loss. Although extensive public health efforts have been dedicated to preventing iron-deficiency anaemia, iron overload is currently more common and possibly more dangerous[2]. The human body has no efficient means of eliminating excess iron. Iron balance is therefore determined by controlled intestinal absorption. Low body stores are associated with more efficient absorption of non-haem iron, the form found in plants. Haem iron, which is found in animal products, is highly absorbed regardless of body iron status, potentially encouraging iron overload. (Haem iron has been implicated in the causation of heart disease and higher iron stores are also associated with cancer as well as poorer response to infection[2]).

According to the Physician's Committee For Responsible Medicine[4], every year 1.1 million Americans are diagnosed with cancer, excluding carcinoma in situ and basal and squamous cell skin cancers and 526,000 Americans die of the disease, accounting for one in every five deaths in the U.S. and 535 billion in direct medical costs. Cancer rates among vegetarians are up to 50 percent below population averages, even after controlling for smoking, body mass index, and socio-economic status. The increased consumption of vegetables and fruits contributes to but does not fully account for, the vegetarians' advantage.

Even more disturbing evidence is also coming to light concerning the development of brain tumours in young children. A study has indicated that a significant risk factor is the amount of contact that the mother may have had with nitrosamines - and this is directly related to maternal consumption of cured meats (Ibid.). Professor Nick Day of the University of Cambridge and the European Prospective Study into Cancer has stated that vegetarians may suffer 40% fewer cancers than the general population. In fact, the World Cancer Research Fund's dietary advice to minimise cancer risk involve reducing the intake of dietary fat and increasing the consumption of fruits, vegetables and whole grains, which is often included in a vegetarian diet (Ibid.).

In the following paragraphs, and to summarise, let us now examine some of the most common types of cancer suffered by Westerners, and its causal relationship with a poor diet as revealed by the PCRM :

OVARIAN CANCER
Recent research into cancer of the ovaries has established a connection between animal fat and cancer. The PCRM say that there was a significant trend towards increasing risk of ovarian cancer with increasing animal fat consumption and one study found that women who consume the most animal fat in their diet run double the risk of contracting ovarian cancer when compared to those who consume the least.

COLON CANCER
As previously mentioned, vegetarians have lower rates of colon cancer than non-vegetarians (Phillips, 1980). Incidence of colon cancer has been strongly linked to the consumption of meat (Armstrong, 1975). Willett (1990) carried out a study of over 88,000 women aged between 34 and 59 years. The study found that women

eating red meat daily ran over twice the risk of developing colon cancer than women eating red meat less than once a month. Reduced incidence of colon cancer in vegetarians may be attributed to dietary differences which include increased fibre intake, increased consumption of fruit and vegetables, and decreased intake of total fat and saturated fat.

The mechanism by which a vegetarian diet is protective against colon cancer is unclear and a great deal of research is being carried out in this area. It has been suggested that secondary bile acids are carcinogens, which may play an important role in colon cancer. These are derived by bacterial metabolism from primary bile acids made in the liver and secreted into the intestine. Vegetarians have lower levels of secondary bile acids than non-vegetarians (Turjiman, 1984). The differences in bacterial populations between the intestines of vegetarians and non-vegetarians may also be important. Bacterial flora in vegetarians has been shown to possess reduced ability to transform bile acids into potential carcinogens([4]).

The role of dietary fibre in prevention of colon cancer may also be important, as was first noted in 1971 when it was suggested that the high incidence of colon cancer in Western countries was linked to low fibre diets. Other dietary components associated with high fibre foods have also been implicated as having protective effects.

BREAST CANCER
Evidence also suggests that a vegetarian diet is protective against breast cancer (Phillips, 1975 cited in [4]). This may be due to the increased fibre and reduced fat intake of vegetarian diets. Vegetarian diets can alter the levels of circulating sex hormones which may have a beneficial effect. Fibre is thought to be protective by modifying circulating oestrogen levels. Studies of adolescent girls have shown the age of menarche (onset of menstruation) to be delayed in vegetarians (Sabate, 1992 cited in Ibid.). A later age of menarche is believed to lower the risk of breast cancer in adult life. (Other studies relating to the links between meat-consumption and breast cancer have already been reported).

There is also evidence to show that Japanese women who eat meat daily have more than eight times the risk of breast cancer compared to poorer women who rarely consume meat([2]).

PROSTRATE CANCER

At one time, talking about prostate cancer was almost a taboo subject and, according to Dr Barnard and A. R. Hogan([5]), that ignorance cost many men their lives. Nowadays though, thanks in part to the willingness of celebrities such as Charlton Heston to go public, awareness of diagnostic methods, etc. have risen sharply. Many men may assume prostate problems are just a part of growing older. Maybe a man starts waking up five or six times a night needing to go to the toilet and, concerned that it could be something serious, he decides to go in for a blood test. Dr Barnard and Hogan argue that what he probably won't be told is how vegetarian meals constitute much better choices to keep the man's cancer odds as low as possible. As with all too many health problems, prevention and alternative methods in overcoming disease still do not get mentioned much; especially the important food factor.

Prostate cancer occurs much less often in Asia than in the United States and Europe, where the average man consumes much more meat, dairy and eggs. A Hong Kong man, for example, is only half as likely as a Swedish man to develop the disease, and only one-eighth as likely to die from it. Not coincidentally, men in Hong Kong eat much less animal fare than Swedes do. The typical Swedish man's diet makes his body fertile soil in which weed-like cancer cells can spread like wildfire (Ibid.).

In another article by the PCRM, entitled 'Diet and Prostate Cancer'([6]), they argue that scientific evidence clearly shows that diet has an important influence on prostate cancer risk. Reduced fat intake helps avert testosterone excesses. Men consuming high-fat diets typically have elevated levels of testosterone in their blood which can over-stimulate the cells of the prostate, increasing cancer risk.

An additional cancer risk relates to a protein in the bloodstream called insulin-like growth factor-I (IGF-I). Although a certain amount of IGF-I in the blood is normal, high levels are linked to increased cancer risk. IGF-I plays a role in cell growth among other functions, and test-tube experiments show that IGF-I encourages cancer cell growth. Diet has a strong influence on IGF-I. In general, excess intake of calories or proteins increases the amount of IGF-I in the blood (Ibid.).

Seventh-day Adventist men have only one-third the prostate cancer risk of other men, and data suggests that the earlier a vegetarian diet is adopted, the lower the risk. Dietary factors may influence not only prostate cancer incidence, but also how quickly it changes from a small growth causing no clinical problems to an advancing, spreading tumour. The prevalence of latent cancers (small growths causing no symptoms) varies somewhat from one country to another, the lowest rates being in Singapore (thirteen percent) and Hong Kong (fifteen percent), and the highest in Sweden (thirty-one percent)[6].

Dr Barnard argues that vegetarians have much lower rates of prostate cancer (and of other cancers, heart disease, stroke, high blood pressure and several other major illnesses). Evidence suggests they also have far less risk of cancer progression if cancer cells do get a foothold. As with any change for the good, the earlier the change is carried out, the better. But foods affect more than just who gets cancer and who does not. They can also ameliorate or exacerbate the course of the disease, once it has started and can affect whether it may recur. Dr Barnard concludes that prostate cancer can indeed be ruthless, but with the right diet Mr. Heston and millions of other men can boost their winning odds[5]. He states that the most important message is that, whilst consumption of meat and dairy products appear to increase cancer risk, diets rich in vegetables and fruits cut the risk, giving men more control over their health than they might otherwise have had[6].

OTHER CANCERS
Studies have shown vegetarians to suffer less from various other cancers. Mills[4] studied the incidence of prostate cancer amongst 14,000 Seventh Day Adventists and found a relationship between

increased risk and increasing animal product consumption. Mills also found pancreatic cancer to be associated with the consumption of animal products. Increasingly, the consumption of fruit, vegetables and pulses was shown to have a protective effect. Also, Rao found a vegetarian diet to be protective against oesophagal cancer (Ibid.). Studies have also shown vegetarians to have a lower incidence of lung cancer. This can be largely attributed to vegetarians tending to be non-smokers. High consumption of fruit has also shown to be protective against lung cancer (Ibid.).

The Diamonds[1], from their extensive studies, argue that **animal products cause cancer, absolutely no doubt about it.** The issue is just how much. If animal products were entirely removed from our diet, cancer (other than smoking-related cancer) would cease to be a problem. Due to their high fat, high cholesterol, low-fibre content, animal products cause cancer, e.g. cancer of the colon, breast, liver, kidneys, prostate, testicles, uterus and ovaries. They argue that, after President Regan's difficulties with cancer of the colon, all of a sudden, *everyone* became interested in the links between diet and cancer, and now organisations such as the National Cancer Institute and the American Cancer Society are finally pointing out that this link does indeed exist - that colon cancer can indeed be *prevented* by 'a good diet'.

Dr Julian Whitaker argues that he looks upon cancer in the same way that he looks upon heart disease, arthritis, high blood pressure, or even obesity, for that matter, in that by dramatically strengthening the body's immune system through diet and exercise, the body can rid itself of the cancer, just as it does in other degenerative diseases. Consequently, he argues that he wouldn't have chemo-therapy and radiation because he's not interested in therapies that cripple the immune system, and virtually ensure failure for the majority of cancer patients[7].

Therefore, the case against meat is looking increasingly grim and the case in favour of an flesh-free, high fresh fruit and vegetable content diet is looking better and better. I'm not sure whether our governments and food producers will ever come clean and actually encourage us to stop eating suspect foods and to start eating healthily (however, it might be that the drug industry make far too much money on the ailing public to consider such a thing). However, the American Dietetic Association came the closest that perhaps any official body has ever come to doing this when it gave this official statement: "The American Dietetic Association recognises that a growing body of scientific evidence supports a positive relationship between the consumption of a plant-based diet and the incidence of certain diseases" (cited in [2]).

But for now, it's over to **YOU,** because if others won't take the right decisions to look after your health, then no-one else is going to....

LEUKAEMIA

Leukaemia is the over-production of white blood cells to contend with toxic materials in the blood, due to the by-products of protein breakdown. As you are probably aware, leukaemia is a type of blood cancer and, as such, the causes (a meat-based diet) would inevitably be the same as for the causes of cancer (above). Dr Paul Kouchakoff discovered, in his extensive experiments, that cooked meat causes a tremendous proliferation of white blood cells in the bloodstream - the increase is 2-4 times that of normal proliferation! The body produces white blood cells in order to surround toxic particles and to escort them to the nearest exit point, usually the kidneys[7].

As already covered in a previous chapter, **leukaemia is always associated with an extremely high amount of uric acid in the blood.** Uric acid is an inevitable by-product of meat consumption, as mentioned in the first chapter. In fact, animal products are approximately 15% uric acid in the first place![8]

CHAPTER THIRTEEN: DIABETES

Diabetes Mellitus is a disease in which the body is unable to control the amount of sugar in the blood because the mechanism which converts sugar to energy is no longer functioning properly, and an estimated 30 million people suffer with it worldwide. Normally the food you eat is gradually broken down and converted to glucose (blood sugar), the source of energy for all your body's functions. The conversion of glucose into energy requires insulin, a hormone produced in the pancreas. Insulin is released into your system in order to control the level of glucose in the blood, especially to prevent your blood sugar level from climbing too high. In diabetics, there is either a shortage of insulin, or the available insulin does not function as it should due to the pancreas being clogged up. In fact, a high-fat diet can cause the cells to be so blocked that insulin can't be retrieved. The result is that glucose is not converted into energy, but builds up in the blood and eventually spills over into the urine. This is often one of the first signs of diabetes. Therefore, though there is an abundance of glucose in the blood, the body is still deprived of the energy it needs (because it has not been converted to energy) and so the liver begins to produce yet more glucose to meet demands. Soon the body's stores of fat and protein begin to break down in another attempt to supply more glucose. This begins a chain of events within the body that can eventually cause severe health problems, even death. In the UK alone, approximately 20,000 people die prematurely of diabetes-related problems each year[1].

There are two main classifications of diabetes (Ibid.): Maturity-Onset Diabetes – non-insulin-dependent type. This type experiences the basic symptoms of thirst, hunger, fatigue and frequent urination. In this type, dietary controls are much more effective. Juvenile Onset Diabetes – this is the insulin dependent type. Those who develop diabetes under the age of 40 years are most likely to suffer the more severe, insulin-dependent type. Children are almost always insulin dependent. This type produces very little or no insulin.

Diabetes is a serious disorder and, unfortunately, its incidence is increasing – in Britain an estimated 60,000 new cases are diagnosed each year. Further, the number of children diagnosed as diabetic has doubled in the past twenty years and this appears to be a worldwide trend([1]). However, there are simple and effective ways in which a person may prevent or reverse the onset of diabetes or minimise its erosion of health (namely by dietary adjustments). **Studies of Seventh-day Adventists, about half of whom are vegetarians, have shown that the prevalence of diagnosed diabetes was 90 percent higher in non-vegetarian men and 40 percent higher in non-vegetarian women, compared to vegetarians.** Controlling for the differences in body weight reduces, but does not eliminate, the differences in diabetes prevalence. In fact, plant-based diets often reduce or eliminate diabetics' medication intake, and reduce the prevalence of neuropathy and renal damage([2]).

The School of Public Health in Minnesota started a massive study of the subject in 1960, which lasted for 21 years and involved 25,698 adult Americans who were Seventh Day Adventists (SDAs). By analysing the death certificates over the period under study, it was possible to assess the increased risk of dying from a diabetic illness. It showed that **taking *any* meat in the diet increases the risk**, on average by 1.8 times. Light meat-eaters (once or twice per week) compared to non-meat-eaters had a relative risk of 1.4 times. Heavy meat-eaters (6 or more times per week) had a relative risk of 3.8 times as likely to die from diabetic-related illness([1]).

The PCRM quote the following studies([2]):

- Snowdon (1985) found Type II diabetes to be only half as common as a cause of death amongst the largely vegetarian Seventh Day Adventist population as compared to the general population.

- An average vegetarian diet closely matches the British Diabetic Association's recommendations for diabetic patients. Vegetarian diets tend to be high in dietary fibre, which has a beneficial effect on carbohydrate metabolism, lowering blood sugar levels. The leanness of vegetarians also contributes to the reduced incidence of diabetes. Also, diabetes is often associated with raised blood cholesterol levels and a vegetarian diet confers protection against this([1]).

So what might be the cause of diabetes? Well, it could be an excess of carbohydrate foods (refined), but what may also be the cause is a diet rich in animal protein. As we have learned, a high-protein diet causes many degenerative diseases and diabetes is amongst them.

Proteolytic enzymes - present in many raw foods - break down protein. An excess of protein, particularly of animal origin, has been linked to a myriad of degenerative conditions, including diabetes, resulting in visible changes which we call ageing and in a shortened lifespan. Three German physicians called Wendt studied the role of excess protein in the diet. With the aid of electron microscopy they were able to show that excess protein clogs the basement membrane, which is a filter between small blood vessels (capillaries) and cells. When this filter is clean and clear, nutrients and oxygen pass through quickly and efficiently from the blood into the cells where they are needed. Similarly, waste products of cell metabolism pass out of the cell quickly, and do not poison the interior of the cell. However, the more protein your diet contains, especially protein of animal origin, the less efficient this process becomes, due to the clogging of the filter, the basement membrane. This, of course, is the beginning of degeneration, of sluggish cell functioning and auto-intoxification of cells([3]). If this process continues for long enough, the clogging becomes so bad that insoluble protein begins to line the capillary and arterial walls, leading to arteriosclerosis, high blood pressure and adult diabetes. Of course, your cells aren't getting the nutrients and oxygen they need. It's hardly surprising that people with degenerative disease feel so tired. But when you avoid all protein of animal origin and eat all foods in their uncooked, raw state (raw protein is easily assimilated and does not lead to this clogging of the basement membrane), nutrients and oxygen can go straight through into the cells. The basement membrane will become thin and porous again([3]).

On the other hand, a high-protein diet in conjunction with over-

eating, bad food combinations that retard or inhibit digestion, cooked foods, animal fats - in short anything in the diet to which humans, as frugivores, are not biologically equipped to handle always causes the body problems. The pancreas is the first organ to be hit by both the chemicals in food, and its low enzyme content. In the absence of sufficient enzymes necessary for the digestion of food, your pancreas takes the load; it simply must manufacture the enzymes itself, if they are not present in the food. It becomes overworked. Here yet again we see a link between some common degenerative diseases and an enzyme-deficient way of eating - diabetes([4]).

Late onset diabetes is caused by a lifetime of eating animal protein and cooked foods and the pancreatic ducts become clogged and, although insulin is produced, it does not get into the cells of the body where it is needed. Insulin works rather like a key, making cell membranes permeable to energy-giving glucose. Without enough of it, glucose accumulates in the blood and eventually overflows into the urine. As well as having to manage their illness for many years, diabetics are faced with a high risk of heart disease and cancer. Until very recently it was assumed that, because high blood glucose levels are what one is trying to avoid, diabetics should not eat carbohydrates, they should eat lots of protein instead. A high protein/low carbohydrate diet together with insulin injections is the traditional method of controlling the illness. But is it the best method? A high-raw diet, low in protein and requiring no special 'diabetic' foods can, it appears, not only reduce the amount of insulin a person needs, but also, in some cases, eliminate the need for it altogether (Ibid.).

The great Albert Schweitzer was a severe diabetic before he sought the help of the raw food pioneer Dr Max Gerson. Schweitzer was very ill indeed and took huge doses of insulin. Gerson took him off his high protein diet because it was his pancreas that had to supply most of the enzymes needed to digest protein, and poorly digested proteins only create more than their fair share of toxic wastes. Gerson put Schweitzer on a regime of fresh raw vegetables and lots of vegetable and fruit juices, including apple juice, with all its fruit sugar. Ten days later Gerson judged it safe to reduce his patient's insulin by half. A month later Schweitzer needed no insulin at all. His diabetes never returned, and he remained healthy and very active until his death in 1965 at the age of 92 (Ibid.).

More recent evidence that diabetes yields to raw food treatments comes from Dr John Douglas, Head of the Health Improvement Service at the Kaiser-Permanente Medical Centre in Los Angeles. Some of his patient's had been able to stop using insulin altogether, while others had reduced its use to a minimum. One of the star cases, a brittle juvenile diabetic, was weaned off insulin and eventually off oral anti-diabetic drugs as well by a 90-100% raw diet. Douglas does find, however, that some diabetics need to restrict the amount of fresh fruit they eat, because fruit contains a lot of sugar. One patient who failed to respond was found to be eating 18 bananas a day! (Ibid.).

Many people who are overweight, suffer from hypoglycaemia or are borderline diabetics and have difficulty in metabolising carbohydrates properly. Indeed, the kind of fatigue and mental depression that comes from low blood sugar, and has you drinking coffee all day and eating sweet things 'just to keep going', predisposes the development of diabetes. Raw foods can change all that. Their high fibre content has proved itself to be an important factor in normalising carbohydrate metabolism and eliminating food cravings. This is why the standard dietary approach to diabetes is rapidly shifting towards the use of more raw foods. Raw food experts such as Dr John Douglas have found that raw carbohydrates are far better tolerated than cooked ones. They don't cause the addictive craving for more that the hypoglycaemic experiences. Douglas, like the Finish expert A. I. Virtanen, also believes that the enzymes in raw foods play an important part in the way they stimulate weight loss, as they do in the treatment of obesity (Ibid.).

In Nauru, a remote island in the Pacific, the population had never had any cases of diabetes until it suddenly became rich and began to import American style fast food. Now more than 40% of the population over the age of 20 have diabetes. The fact is that diabetes is more common amongst meat-eaters. Meat-eating increases

129

consumption of saturated fats, which may affect insulin sensitivity and also the N-nitroso compounds in meat may be a trigger to the development of diabetes. The massive study, started in 1960 amongst over 25,000 American Seventh Day Adventists, showed that people who ate meat run twice the risk of dying from a diabetes-related cause. The correlation between meat consumption and diabetes was found to be particularly strong in males. (The study was carefully designed to eliminate confusion arising from confounding factors such as over or underweight or amount of physical activity). **The study shows that eating any meat increases the risk by 1.8 times[1].**

According to the Diabetes Epidemiology Research International to the British Medical Journal, between 60 and 95% of cases of insulin-dependent diabetes can be prevented. They believe that environmental factors are largely responsible for the increase in diabetes, claiming that genetic factors could not be responsible for such a large increase over a very short time period. They reported that **diet was the most significant and controllable environmental cause[1].**

Cox states that The American Diabetes Association suggests that diabetics eat a diet in which carbohydrates make up about 60% of their total calorie intake; from unrefined, complex and high-fibre foods. There is an emphasis on reducing saturated fats and cholesterol and replacing these with monounsaturated fats such as olive oil and they recommend protein intake be moderate. This is because diabetes is more common amongst meat-eaters, and saturated fats increase insulin sensitivity. Also, the N-nitroso compounds in meat may actually be a trigger to the development of diabetes[1].

Diabetics are particularly vulnerable to high levels of fat in their blood, and meat is a prime source of saturated fat. There may also be a problem with excess protein consumption too. Several clinical studies have now shown that a low-protein diet can also help to slow down the decline in kidney function that can occur in diabetics (Ibid.).

In an article entitled "Can a Vegan Diet Cure Diabetes?" (5), Andrew Nicholson, M.D. writes that diabetes is not necessarily a one-way street. Early studies suggest that people with diabetes can improve and, in some cases, even cure themselves of the disease by switching to an unrefined, vegan diet. Since none of the previous studies included a comparison group, the Diabetes Action and Research Education Foundation provided a grant to the PCRM to perform a carefully-controlled test. Working with Georgetown University, they compared two different diets: a high-fibre, low-fat vegan diet, and the more commonly used American Diabetes Association (ADA) diet.

Dr Nicholson says that in the study, people with non-insulin-dependent diabetes and their spouses or partners were invited to follow one of the two diets for three months. The vegan meals were made from unrefined vegetables, grains, beans, and fruits, with no refined ingredients such as vegetable oil, white flour or white pasta. The comparison (ADA) diet contained somewhat more plant-based ingredients than the average American diet, but still relied upon the conventional chicken and fish recipes.

The results were extremely encouraging. One participant said he was amazed at how powerful the vegan diet was right from the beginning. His blood sugars and weight just started falling off! Some subjects were pleasantly surprised at how well they adapted to the experimental diet. One said, "If anyone had told me twelve weeks ago that I would be satisfied with a totally vegetarian diet, I would not have believed it." Another participant said that he was no longer on medication for diabetes or any medication for blood pressure. He said "So, actually, it's been a very, very positive result for me". Some found unexpected benefits, such as one participant who said "My asthma has really improved. I'm not taking as much asthma medicine because I can breathe better. The overall mental outlook on how I feel about myself as a diabetic is much more hopeful now, as I am self-sufficient with a diet that makes sense for me."

The vegan group clearly had the leading edge in many of the results. Fasting blood sugars decreased fifty-nine percent more in the vegan group than in the ADA group. Also, whilst the vegan group needed less medication to control their blood sugars, the ADA group needed just as much medicine as before. The vegans were not only taking less medication, they were also in better control. The vegan group lost nearly sixteen pounds on average, and cholesterol levels also dropped more substantially than in the ADA group.

Diabetes can cause serious damage to the kidneys, resulting in protein loss in the urine. Several of the subjects already had significant protein loss at the beginning of the study, and the ADA group did not improve in this respect. In fact, their protein losses actually worsened somewhat over the twelve weeks of the study. The vegan group, on the other hand, had a large reduction in protein losses.

So, again we find studies linking another form of degenerative disease - diabetes - with the consumption of flesh foods. Because flesh foods are alien to our physiology, our bodies are placed under great strain when we consume this type of food. On a meat-free diet however, again there is a greatly reduced incidence of this type of disease, and even a reversal of this condition, when placed on a raw food diet and, particularly under the competent supervision of a practitioner who is knowledgeable about the necessary precautions that must be taken in the care of diabetes, i.e. a practitioner who has been trained in Natural Hygiene.

CHAPTER FOURTEEN:
HEART DISEASE AND HYPERTENSION

Cardiovascular disease is the major cause of mortality in Britain, being responsible for around 50% of all deaths. The majority of these deaths are from coronary heart disease. Vegetarians suffer markedly lower mortality from coronary heart disease, as compared to non-vegetarians. This reduced risk may be related to the lower blood cholesterol levels of vegetarians.

According to Cox, as early as 1961, The Journal of the American Medical Association reported that "a vegetarian diet can prevent 90-97% of heart diseases (thromboembolic disease and coronary occlusions)". In fact, in recent years scientific studies have shown that a vegan diet can heal the damage inflicted on clogged arteries([2]).

A Japanese study from the National Cancer Centre Research Institute in Tokyo tracked the health of 122,261 people over 16 years. Two lifestyles emerged from this study, one being very low risk and the other being very high risk lifestyles. The high risk being smoking, drinking, meat-consumption and no green vegetables and the low-risk being the opposite. Deaths from all causes were elevated by 1.53 times amongst those who smoked, drank and ate meat. The scientists found that their risk of heart disease was 1.88 times higher and the risk of any kind of cancer was 2.49 times higher. However, **they found that simply by adding one factor – meat consumption – to an otherwise healthy lifestyle had a serious effect on mortality** (Ibid.).

The PCRM([1]) describe the following studies in their 1995 News Report:

- Burr and Butiand (1988) found vegetarians to suffer significantly lower mortality from heart disease than even health conscious non-vegetarians. Mortality from ischaemic heart disease was 57% lower in vegetarians than the general population, and 18% lower than in non-vegetarians following a healthy lifestyle. Deaths due to cerebrovascular disease were 43% lower in vegetarians, compared with the general population.

- The Coronary Artery Risk Development in Young Adults (CARDIA) Study examined diet in relation to health in over 5,000 young adults aged 18 to 30. Vegetarians were found to have greatly improved cardiovascular fitness and a lower risk of heart disease (Slattery, 1991).

- An eleven-year study of 1,900 German vegetarians found mortality from cardiovascular disease to be 61% lower in male vegetarians and 44% lower in female vegetarians than the general population. For ischaemic heart disease, mortality was reduced still further, to only one-third of that expected (Claude-Chang, 1992).

- The protective effects of a vegetarian diet are believed to be related to the lower blood cholesterol levels seen in vegetarians. Repeated studies have demonstrated the low blood cholesterol levels of vegetarians (Resnicow, 1991). High blood cholesterol is a primary risk factor in heart disease. Significantly, vegetarians have lower levels of low-density-lipoprotein (LDL) cholesterol. This is the cholesterol fraction particularly associated with heart disease.

- The California Lifestyle Heart Trial has indicated that a low fat vegetarian diet, together with other lifestyle changes such as exercise and stress management, can in fact reverse the progress of heart disease, by reducing cholesterol plaques in coronary arteries (Ornish, 1990).

So what is it that makes meat so harmful to the circulatory system? The probable reason is that the fats of animal flesh, such as cholesterol, do not break down in the human body. These fats begin to line the walls of our blood vessels. When there is a process of continual accumulation, the opening inside the vessels gets smaller and smaller as the years go by, leading to arteriosclerosis which places a tremendous burden on the heart to pump the blood through clogged and constricted vessels. As a result of this, high blood pressure, strokes and heart attacks readily occur.

According to the Diamonds[3], cholesterol is a substance unique to animals and humans. It is secreted by the liver and is necessary for many functions of the body. The human body secretes about 2,000 milligrams of cholesterol daily, and the body uses it in *all* of its tissues. The body will secrete its needs daily whether or not you take any in with food, because *only its own* can be utilised. However, cholesterol taken in via the diet is a severe health hazard. Animal products are *very* high in fat, *very* high in cholesterol and *very* low in fibre. Animal protein raises blood cholesterol and saturated fats from animal products raise cholesterol levels and increase your chances of dying of heart disease.

Amazingly, the first clinical sign of someone suffering a heart attack was recorded as recently as 1912! Until then it seems to have been rare, for they were not recorded. Today, heart disease is the commonest cause of death in the Western world. Britain is the 'heart attack capital' of the world.

In 1970, both America and Australia had higher rates of death from heart disease than the UK. However, since then the impacts of health-promoting measures in both countries have meant that America's death-rate has declined by 55% and Australia's by 51%. Britain, however, has only fallen by 24%. British males are the most vulnerable group in 35-74 year olds. In fact, heart disease is responsible for one in three deaths amongst males and one in four amongst females. After cancer, it is the leading cause of premature death amongst women[2].

In 1990, the Editor-in-Chief of the American Journal of Cardiology wrote:

> *Although human beings eat meat, we are not natural carnivores. We were intended to eat plants, fruits and starches! No matter how much fat carnivores eat, they do not develop atherosclerosis. Its virtually impossible, for example, to produce atherosclerosis in a dog even when 100g of cholesterol and 120g of butter fat are added to its meat ration (this is approximately 200 times the average amount that human*

beings in the USA eat each day!). In contrast, herbivores rapidly develop atherosclerosis if they are fed foods, namely fat and cholesterol, intended for natural carnivores.... Thus, although we think we are one and we act as if we are one, human beings are not natural carnivores. When we kill animals or eat them, they end up killing us because their flesh, which contains cholesterol and saturated fat, was never intended for human beings, who are natural herbivores (cited in Cox, [2]).

Indeed, Dr David Ryde (Ibid.), an English family doctor, reported the following: "My first was a patient with severe angina. His condition had been deteriorating for about five years and he'd been into hospital, was taking all the medication and so on. But his condition was, quite frankly, almost terminal. It was really a pitiful sight to see him struggle to walk the few yards from the car to the surgery. Now a person in such a desperate state will listen and they will try anything." Dr Ryde suggested a vegan diet, and reported the following: "Just one month later, he could walk one mile. Three months later he could walk four miles, while carrying shopping. It used to take him a quarter of an hour to climb three flights of steps" his daughter told me. "Now he's up in a few seconds!".

That was Dr Ryde's first success, and it encouraged him to go on to treat many other patients in this way. One case had blood pressure of 185/120 and, upon trying a vegan diet, this came down to 115/75 and she felt fantastic (anti-hypertensive medication often leaves patients feeling exhausted).

Dr Ryde argues: "I've seen results such as these in my patients too often to attribute them to coincidence. Really this kind of treatment has no side-effects, and the benefits are so worthwhile, that there's no reason not to try it."

In 1978 Dr Roland Phillips, one of America's most respected Epidemiologists, published his study in the American Journal of Clinical Nutrition. His study was again of Seventh Day Adventists in America, and his sample was massive: 25,000 people. The study took six years and the SDA's were compared against – wait for it – the average meat-eating population for the area. The study concluded

136

that the SDA's risk of dying from coronary heart disease was far lower than normal. For every 100 males who died from heart disease, 26 SDA males had died – that's about one quarter of the risk. Amongst females, the risk was one third. Dr Phillips and his team had considered the possibility that the results were attributable to smoking, so they next compared deaths from heart disease amongst SDAs and a representative group of non-smokers, as studied by the American Cancer Society. If the hypothesis that smoking was the answer were true, then the death rates would be the same. But they weren't – in fact, they were a long way off! The SDAs had only half the risk of dying from heart disease, when compared to non-smokers (people identified as *never having smoked* by the American Cancer Society). **This study took 20 years in all to perform and provided the first ever scientific proof that the more meat you eat, the more at risk from heart disease you become.**

Also, in The Encyclopaedia for Vegetarian Living([2]), a study is included of 4,671 British non-meat-eaters. This study tracked their health for seven years and also found very similar conclusions. For heart disease, the male death rate was only 44% and the female rate was 41% of the norm, compared to the general population.

According to Dr Neal Barnard of the PCRM([5]), what many people still don't know, and their doctors seldom tell them, is that the very best way of eating right for your heart and the rest of your body means adopting a plant-based diet. He argues that a December 1999 article in the 'Journal of the American Medical Association' proves again that a low-fat vegetarian diet, along with mild exercise, no smoking and reduced stress, is the best bet for heart disease patients.

Dean Ornish, M.D., reported on a five-year follow-up of patients on his popular plan for reversing heart disease, compared with patients on the chicken and fish diet recommended by the American Heart Association (AHA). The majority of those following the AHA guidelines got progressively worse, while those who made intensive changes got progressively better.

Plant foods contain no cholesterol. Animal products always do. For every one percent increase in cholesterol levels, heart attack risks rises by two percent. For every 100 milligrams of cholesterol in the daily diet; the typical amount in a four-ounce serving of either beef or chicken, one's cholesterol level typically zooms up five points. (As mentioned, unlike fat, cholesterol concentrates in 'lean meat'.) Dr Barnard argues that the soap-opera ads on television go on about a waxy build-up on your kitchen floors, but what should really worry you is a dangerous, wax-like cholesterol plaque build-up inside your blood vessels. This hardening of the arteries can interrupt the smooth flow of blood and trigger chest pains (angina), blood clots, and heart attacks.

The PCRM state([1]), that an estimated 1 million Americans suffer heart attacks each year, 45% of whom are under age 65. Heart disease accounts for $40 billion in annual health care costs. Ovo-lacto-vegetarians have about one-half to three quarters the risk of dying of heart disease, compared to non-vegetarians, even after controlling for other lifestyle factors. Cholesterol levels are much lower in vegetarians, and vegetarian diets reduce serum cholesterol levels to a much greater degree than is achieved with the National Cholesterol Education Program Step Two diet.

Dr. David Jenkins, Canadian Research Chair in Metabolism and Nutrition at the University of Toronto and St. Michael's Hospital([7]) believes that the less we eat like our ancestors, the more likely we'll succumb to heart disease. The possibility that our dietary requirements are programmed in our genes - the blueprint in every cell that controls all body processes - is a notion that has intrigued Jenkins for some time. "Our genes only differ from our great ape cousins by 3 per cent," says Jenkins. If our genes are ancient, our diet most certainly is not. Today's fast fare of processed, refined foods provides only a fraction of the vitamins, minerals and fibre than it once did. Does this mean that the foods we eat and the diseases that plague us are out of sync with our evolutionary origins? According to Jenkins, maybe so. He recently studied the effects of primeval diets on blood cholesterol levels in healthy volunteers and found dramatic effects.

138

Participants followed three evolutionary diets, each one for two weeks at a time. The oldest, the Great Ape Diet, consisted of fruits, vegetables, leafy greens and nuts, but no starch or animal foods. Volunteers ate plenty of vegetable protein, little fat and virtually no cholesterol. The next diet represented the Neolithic period, some 10,000 years ago. With the advent of agriculture, our Stone Age ancestors ate starchy foods like oats, legumes and other grains. Participants ate what resembled a low fat Mediterranean diet - whole grains, fruits, vegetables, beans, olives and low fat dairy products were daily foods. Introducing starch into the diet meant eating fewer fruits and vegetables, and as a result, daily fibre intake, although still very high, dropped by more than half. If you've seen a dietitian for high cholesterol, you might be familiar with Jenkins' third diet. It adhered to contemporary cholesterol lowering guidelines - low in total and saturated fat, and no more than 200 milligrams of cholesterol per day. Compared to the diets of our ancestors, these meals were considerably lower in fruits, vegetables and dietary fibre (25 grams/day). To Jenkins' surprise, after one week on the Great Ape Diet, participants' LDL (bad) cholesterol levels dropped by 33 per cent, the same magnitude you'd see with cholesterol lowering drugs called statins. The Stone Age diet was about two-thirds as good, while the modern diet had only a modest effect on blood cholesterol. Jenkins attributes these heart-healthy effects to three key ingredients - soluble fibre, vegetable protein, and naturally occurring compounds called plant sterols - all abundant in the ape diet. "If you consider that 50 per cent of middle-aged men might benefit from taking a statin [drug]" says Jenkins, "these evolutionary diets give people an option"[7].

HYPERTENSION
Hypertension is the medical term for high blood pressure. It has been proven time and time again that the high fat content of animal products (meat and dairy products, etc.) contribute to high blood pressure and that as saturated fat is lowered in the diet, blood pressure tends to go down[3].

139

The PCRM([6]) report that as early as 1917 doctors noticed hospitalized patients had less hypertension when they did not eat meat. In 1926, researchers reported a significant rise in blood pressure among vegetarian college students within two weeks of adding meat to their diets and a 1930 German study found that those who avoided meat had lower blood pressure than meat-eaters, regardless of their ages.

Dr Barnard says that high blood pressure (or hypertension) adds to the risk of heart attacks. Even without lessening one's salt intake, eating a low-fat, high-fibre vegetarian diet can lower blood pressure by ten percent, for reasons not yet clear. (However, he advises that leaving the salt shaker alone is also smart.) In addition, vegetarians store less iron, which counters the strong link between excessive iron and heart disease (Ibid.).

In 1983, a study published in the journal 'Nutrition Report International' showed that vegetarians did not experience the age-related blood pressure rises seen in meat-eaters of similar age, sex and weight. In fact, the longer they avoided meat, the lower their blood pressures. Also in 1983, the 'American Journal of Clinical Nutrition' reported that blood pressures exceeding 160/95 occurred in thirteen times as many non-vegetarians as vegetarians. Carefully designed research that adjusted for age, obesity, heart rate, weight change, exercise and other factors, found that both systolic and diastolic blood pressure drops when meat-eaters follow meat-free diets. Lowered blood pressure results from going vegetarian, regardless of whether a person's blood pressure was initially normal, high or very high. Even extra weight (as much as twenty percent above average) and lack of exercise make little difference.

For years, medical science has focused on eliminating or controlling immediate causes of hypertension, leaving the underlying causes largely unexplored. Efforts to limit salt intake, lose weight and increase exercise do help, but with so many people still succumbing to the condition, we obviously need a deeper solution and an avoidance of eating animal flesh is that solution.

More than eight decades of mostly ignored research shows the power of a diet change to lower blood pressure and limit heart disease risks. Delicious meals consisting of fruits, vegetables and legumes offer a bounty of health-promoting nutrients. Rich in potassium, which lowers blood pressure, a vegetarian diet contain less salt and fat than animal products, and low cholesterol. Indeed, a vegetarian diet does much more than lower a patient's blood pressure (Ibid.).

According to the PCRM([1]), an estimated sixty-three million Americans have high blood pressure, nearly half of whom are unaware that they have it. The associated annual health care costs total more than $5.12 thousand million. The prevalence of hypertension among vegetarians is about one-third to one-half that of non-vegetarians, and adopting a vegetarian diet significantly lowers blood pressure in both normal and hypertensive individuals. The effect is independent of changes in body weight and salt or fat intake, and is not fully accounted for by the presence or absence of any nutrient or group of nutrients. Hypertension, or high blood pressure, can contribute to heart disease, strokes and kidney failure.

It is, of course, well-known that salt does cause high blood pressure and it should be noted that many meat products contain salt, ranging from high to low amounts. This may be through sodium nitrate which, as mentioned, is used as a preservative to stop flesh turning a sickly grey colour which is the invevitable colour of decaying flesh to turn or from sodium chloride (table salt) being directly added to the meat. Processed foods also contain salt (often quite a lot). Even sea salt, touted as a healthy option is harmful to our health, and the body will beg for water in an attempt to dilute the poison! Therefore, all foods which contain *added* salt, sea salt or salt water should be avoided([4]).

Recently, several large, well-designed studies have shown a clear association between homocysteine levels and heart attack and stroke. Homocysteine builds up in some people to detrimental effect. Not only does meat and dairy consumption raise cholesterol, it also raises homocysteine levels, which is now widely seen as a separate risk marker for heart disease. It has also been shown that vitamins and

141

supplements are not as effective as diet in lowering homocysteine levels. This led the American Heart Association last year to make the following statement: Fresh fruits and vegetables, rather than vitamin supplements, are the best line of defense against raised homocysteine levels, an indicator of heart diseases.

We have now come to the end of specific disease chapters, and I hope that it is now apparent that adopting a strict vegetarian, high raw-food diet is a very good insurance policy for protecting against many forms of ill-health. Of course, there are other contributing causes of the major diseases which human's commonly suffer from, for instance, stress, pollution, lack of sunshine, lack of exercise, etc., however, diet has been proven time and time again to be a very big factor in the causation of most degenerative disease, and is usually the very thing that most people do wrong!

CHAPTER FIFTEEN: OTHER HUMAN CONDITIONS AND THEIR RELATIONSHIP TO MEAT CONSUMPTION

The following human conditions and diseases have been proven in studies to be less prevalent in vegetarian people:

OBESITY

Vegetarians are generally leaner than non-vegetarians and their weights are generally closer to desirable levels. The British Medical Association (1986) has stated that vegetarians have lower rates of obesity. This may be due partly to vegetarians being more aware of their diet and of what a healthy diet should constitute. Obesity is a major contributor to many serious illnesses. Vegetarians are, on average about ten percent leaner than meat-eaters, and the adoption of such a diet typically results in substantial weight loss[1].

DIVERTICULAR DISEASE

Diverticular disease affects the colon and symptoms include lower abdominal pain and disturbed bowel habit. It occurs frequently in Western countries, where intake of dietary fibre is low. Gear (1979) found diverticular disease to be less frequent in vegetarians, twelve percent of vegetarians had diverticular disease, compared with thirty-three percent of non-vegetarians. This is thought to be due to the increased fibre of vegetarian diets (Ibid.).

GALLBLADDER DISEASE

Every year, more than 500,000 Americans undergo gallbladder surgery at an estimated annual cost of fifty-three thousand million dollars. Vegetarians have about one-third the prevalence of a history of gallbladder disease and related surgery, compared to meat-eaters (Ibid.).

GALLSTONES

Gallstones are composed of cholesterol, bile pigments and calcium salts. They form in the gall bladder and can cause severe pain. A study of over seven hundred and fifty women found the incidence of gallstones to be less frequent in vegetarians. Twenty-five percent of non-vegetarians compared with twelve percent of vegetarians had gallstones. After controlling for age and body weight, non-vegetarians were found to have a relative risk of gallstones almost twice that of the vegetarians (Pixiey, 1985). Vegetarians are leaner, and consume more dietary fibre and less dietary cholesterol, all of which is believed to protect against gallstone formation ([1]).

KIDNEY STONES
Kidney stones form in the kidney and can cause considerable pain when passing down the urinary tract. Prevalence of kidney stones is lower in vegetarians (Peacock, 1969). A high intake of animal protein increases the urinary loss of calcium and oxalate, known risk factors in kidney stone formation. Meat is also high in purines which leads to increased uric acid in the urine. Urinary uric acid is also a risk factor for kidney stones([1]).

APPENDICITIS
The Oxford Vegetarian Study found that people who do not eat meat have a 50% lower risk of requiring an emergency appendectomy than those who do (Appleby, 1995 cited in [1]).

PRE-MENSTRUAL SYNDROME
In an article entitled 'Nutritional Factors in Menstrual Pain and Pre-menstrual Syndrome'([2]), Neal D. Barnard, M.D argues that disorders of menstrual function can be taxing and sometimes even disabling. In most cases, there is no identifiable cause, however, for some women, the pain is a symptom of endometriosis (a condition in which cells that normally line the uterus have ended up in the abdominal cavity), adenomyosis (the existence of islands of uterine lining cells deep within the uterine muscle), fibroids (the presence of over-grown muscle cells in the wall of the uterus), or other conditions.

Nutritional factors appear to play an important role in managing menstrual pain. Pre-menstrual syndrome includes feelings of moodiness, tension or irritability, as well as physical symptoms such as water retention. Like menstrual pain, it appears to be influenced by nutrition. Dr Barnard states that one of the treatments they have been testing is the use of a very-low-fat, vegetarian diet because when it is properly followed, it has the very helpful effect of reducing the amount of oestrogen in the blood, sometimes to a striking degree. For some individuals at least, diets that avoid animal products and keep vegetable oils to a bare minimum cause a marked reduction in menstrual pain, presumably because of the diet's effect on hormones.

There are several reasons why this diet affects hormones. First of all, reducing the amount of fat in your diet reduces the amount of oestrogen in your blood. This appears to be true for all fats; animal fats and vegetable oils. Second, plant products contain fibre (roughage), which tends to carry oestrogens out of the body. The liver filters oestrogens out of the blood and sends them down a small tube, called the bile duct, into the digestive tract. There, fibre from grains, beans, vegetables and fruits soaks up oestrogens like a sponge. Of course, the amount of fibre in your diet is reduced when you have yoghurt, chicken breast, eggs or any other animal products because fibre comes only from plants. Without adequate fibre, the oestrogens in your digestive tract end up being reabsorbed back into the bloodstream. In addition to individual reports that a low-fat vegetarian diet can cause dramatic reductions in menstrual pain, vegetarians also have fewer ovulatory disturbances (Ibid.).

In conclusion, the diet that has been extremely helpful in individuals excludes animal products completely and also keeps vegetable oils very low. Dr Barnard states that in his experience the diet must be followed closely in order for it to work. This means that no animal products at all, not even skimmed milk or eggs, should be consumed. It also means keeping vegetable oils to a bare minimum in the diet, as mentioned. Even though olive oil or peanut butter are better than chicken fat or beef fat when it comes to cholesterol levels, the effect on hormones is what we are concerned about here, and all fats; animal fats and vegetable oils have to be avoided because they all cause extra oestrogen to be made by your body. So, in addition to keeping animal products out of the diet, it is important to avoid oily salad dressings, chips, crisps, butter, margarine, cooking oils, and the shortening that is in many biscuits and pastries. It also appears to be important to make this change for the entire month, not just before your period. Some people also note that other problems, such as migraines are less common with this kind of diet.

Dr Barnard points out that different kinds of fats act differently in your body. For instance, animal fat contains a great deal of saturated fat, which is the kind of fat that is solid at room temperature, while vegetable oils contain more unsaturated fats, which are liquids. Fats influence the production of prostaglandins in your body and these natural chemicals are involved in inflammation, pain, muscle contractions, blood vessel constriction and blood clotting. Prostaglandins are suspected of playing a role in menstrual pain, migraines, and gastrointestinal pains. He argues that the best strategy is to keep your diet rich in green leafy vegetables and legumes (beans, peas, and lentils) and to eliminate all meats and other animal products (Ibid.).

MULTIPLE SCLEROSIS
In an article entitled 'Treating Multiple Sclerosis with Diet: Fact or Fraud?', John A. McDougall, M.D.[3] says that most health professionals dismiss the idea that multiple sclerosis (MS), a degenerative disease of the nervous system, might be linked to diet. It seems ridiculous to them that so mysterious a disease may be affected by something so simple. Rather than looking to the kitchen for answers, the medical establishment expects a cure for multiple sclerosis to come from high-tech research that will pinpoint some culprit; a virus, perhaps, or a glitch in the immune system. Nevertheless, McDougall argues that all of the existing scientific evidence points to diet as the most helpful approach.

Multiple sclerosis is the most common degenerative inflammatory neurological disease in the U.S., striking people primarily between the ages of 15 and 55. It is characterised by numerous lesions, areas of damage on the nerve cells of the brain and/or spinal cord. The lesions are replaced by hard scar tissue, causing the nerve cells to stop functioning. The nearly 500,000 Americans with MS suffer recurrent attacks on the nervous system that rob them of various functions and senses. One attack may take a victim's vision; the next may cause loss of bladder control; a few months later, one arm or leg may no longer have strength. After ten years with the disease, half of all MS victims are severely disabled; bed-ridden, wheelchair-bound, or worse.

The present approach to MS is a failure. The powerful medications being used have done little to help. The International Federation of Multiple Sclerosis Societies recently examined one hundred and forty therapies (excluding diet) and concluded that no treatment has been shown to alter the course of the disease. This frightening fact should make researchers eager to consider any approach that has the slightest possibility of improving the health of MS patients.

Multiple sclerosis is common in Canada, the U.S., and Northern Europe, but rare in Africa and Asia. When people migrate from a country of low MS incidence to a country of high incidence (which inevitably changes the way they live and eat), their risk for getting the disease increases. Many studies have investigated the environmental factors that could account for the difference in disease occurrence among various populations. The main factor appears to be the strongest contact we have with our environment: our daily food intake. Although wealthy countries generally have higher rates of MS and less affluent countries have lower ones, there is one exception: Japan. Even though the Japanese live in a modern, industrialised country with all the stress, pollution and smoking habits common to other industrialised nations, their rice-based diet is more characteristic of the foods consumed in poorer nations where MS is less common. Dr McDougall states that the Japanese case provides strong evidence that a diet heavy in animal foods, not other modern scourges, may lay the foundation for MS. Of course, all aspects of a diet filled with rich foods can cause problems, but animal fats; especially those from dairy products; have been the most closely linked to the development of MS.

There is one theory which suggests that feeding cow's milk to infants lays the foundation for nervous system injury later in life. Cow's milk has only one-fifth as much linoleic acid (an essential fatty acid) as human breast milk. Linoleic acid makes up the building blocks for nervous tissues. It may be that children raised on a high animal-fat diet deficient in linoleic acid (as most children are in our society) develop a weaker nervous system that is susceptible to problems as they age. Analysis of brain tissues has shown that people with MS have a higher saturated fat content in their brains than people without the disease. Most likely, the offender is connected to the circulatory system in the brain or spinal cord, because the lesions and scarring characteristic of MS are centred in nerve cells near blood vessels. (For more information on the links between cow's milk and MS please refer to Dairy Products section).

Another theory holds that MS attacks are caused by a decreased supply of blood to the sensitive brain tissues. Dietary fat can have this effect. It enters the bloodstream and coats the blood cells. As a result, the cells stick together, forming clumps that slow the flow of blood to vital tissues. The blood does not form clots (as in the case of strokes), but in many blood vessels the clumping becomes so severe that the flow of blood stops and the overall oxygen content of the blood falls. Tissues deprived of blood and oxygen for long periods of time will die. Could something this simple be a factor in MS?

As an example, let's take a look at the health of people on a fat-restricted diet. During World War II, food was scarce and stress was high in occupied Western Europe. People could no longer afford to eat meat, so they turned instead to the grains and vegetables that once nourished their cows, chickens, and pigs. The result was a dramatic reduction in the intake of animal products and of total fat in the diet. Doctors observed that patients with MS had 2 to 2-1/2 times fewer hospitalisations during the war years!

Roy Swank, M.D., former head of the University of Oregon's neurology department and now a practicing physician at Oregon Health Sciences University, observed that MS patients improved on this forced low-fat diet. In the 1950s, Swank began treating his own patients with such a diet. He got excellent results, so for the next 35 years he treated thousands of MS patients in this way. By any medical standard, his results have been remarkable: patients' conditions improved by as much as 95 percent. Patients fared better if they had detected the disease early and had had few attacks, but even long-

148

time MS sufferers experienced a slowdown of the disease's progression. Originally Swank was most concerned with limiting saturated fat, but over the years he has become more attuned to the dangers of all kinds of fat. His MS diet is now about twenty percent fat by calories. Swank's results are unchallenged by other studies, but instead of advocating a low-fat vegetarian diet for MS patients, many doctors either ignore Swank's work or dismiss it because they think the diet would be too difficult to follow.

When Swank was asked why his studies have largely been ignored by the MS research establishment, he told Dr McDougall, "John, I'm a little guy in this little lab at the university. Their research funds didn't pay for this, so how could it be important?" The important findings which emerged from Swank's research, however, were as follows: The earlier an MS patient adopted a low-fat diet, the better the chance of avoiding deterioration and death from the disease. The death rate was 21 percent for the patients who kept to that low level of fat consumption and who started the diet within three years of diagnosis of the disease. On the other hand, patients consuming more than 25 grams of saturated fat daily had a death rate of 79 percent over the period of the study; nearly half of those deaths were directly due to MS. In fact, Swank has shown that the 8-gram difference in daily intake of saturated fat (which triples the death rate for victims of MS) can mean as little as:

1 oz. pork sausage (10 grams)
1 medium-fat hamburger (14 grams)
3 oz. porterhouse steak (14 grams)
1 oz. cheddar cheese (9 grams)
2 tsp. butter (8 grams)
1 cup whole milk (8 grams)

The findings are clear. To arrest MS, the diet must be as low in saturated fat as possible. This translates into a low-fat vegetarian diet: one of starches, vegetables and fruits; delicious foods containing only five to ten percent total fat. If you skip eggs, dairy products and tropical oils such as coconut or palm kernel oil, you eat virtually no saturated fat. Besides arresting MS, a low-fat vegetarian diet promotes weight loss in the obese, relieves constipation, and cuts the food bill by 40 percent. In fact, this type of diet is in line with recommendations made by other health organisations (including the American Cancer Society, the American Heart Association and the Surgeon General's office) that urge Americans (and other Westerners) to eat less fat, meat and dairy products, whilst adding more whole grains, vegetables and fruits (Ibid.). Dr McDougall points out that he treats his MS patients with a wholefood vegetarian diet with no added oil, eggs or dairy products. He states that he has been very gratified by the results of this dietary treatment, not only because the progress of most of his MS patients' diseases have been halted, but also because their overall health has unquestionably improved. He further adds that everyone knows that MS sufferers need every bit of help they can get.

FOOD POISONING AND PESTICIDE RESIDUES
Over 58,000 cases of food poisoning were reported in 1990 and the actual incidence of food poisoning is estimated to be ten times this figure. Meat, eggs and dairy products are the primary sources of food poisoning. Professor Richard Lacey of the University of Leeds has stated that "More than 95% of food poisoning is derived from meat and poultry products"[1]. Pesticide residues in foods include PCB's and dioxins. These are found in highest concentrations in meat, particularly fish, and dairy products. Studies have shown these toxic chemicals can be passed on from pregnant women to infants during both pregnancy and lactation, and may damage the developing nervous systems. Hall (1992) has stated that a vegetarian diet minimises the risk of contamination[1].

NEPHROTIC SYNDROME
Nephrotic syndrome is a kidney condition involving high levels of protein in the urine which may lead to progressive kidney damage as well as promoting atherosclerosis and heart disease. Studies have shown a low protein vegan diet can be used to reduce the symptoms of nephrotic syndrome (D'Amico, 1992 cited in Ibid.).

ALZHEIMER'S DISEASE

A review of studies published during the past two years sheds significant light on a central risk factor in Alzheimer's - high levels of a blood substance called homocysteine. Homocysteine is an amino acid, and amino acids are the building blocks of proteins. The only source of homocysteine for use in our bodies is that which is formed by the liver after the ingestion of another amino acid, methionine. Methionine is found in protein foods and animal protein contains two to three times the amount of methionine as does plant protein. Researchers say they found serum-homocysteine to be an early and sensitive marker for cognitive impairment. In patients with dysmentia (mild cognitive impairment), no less than 39% had pathological serum-homocysteine levels. The study, conducted in Sweden, not only showed blood levels of homo-cysteine to correlate strongly with Alzheimer's disease - but showed elevated levels of homocysteine were useful in *predicting* who might get Alzheimer's[4]. As you will note from previous chapters, vegetarians have been shown to have a lower level of homocysteine in their bloodstream.

In another study (Ibid.) reported at the World Alzheimer's Congress in July 2000, researchers studied 5,395 individuals aged 55 and over who were free from dementia. After examining subjects in 1993 and again in 1999 researchers reported the following: On average, people who remained free from any form of dementia had consumed higher amounts of beta-carotene, vitamin C, vitamin E and vegetables than the people in the study who developed Alzheimer's disease. The researchers also noted that in this study, family history or the presence of a genetic marker called the ApoE4 allele (both considered risk factors for Alzheimer's) did not alter their findings. In other words, high consumption of vegetables appeared to offset one of the other known risk factors for Alzheimer's.

So How Can You Lower Your Risk of Alzheimer's?

In addition to avoiding dietary and cosmetic sources of aluminium, maintain a low homocysteine level by greatly reducing consumption of the homocystein-producing amino acid methionine - through avoiding flesh foods and products. If you're on one of those high-protein fad diets, just be aware that along with the extra pounds you may temporarily lose, you may just lose your mind too by setting the later stage for becoming an Alzheimer's casualty. We already know from a 1993 study that subjects who ate meat, including poultry and fish, were more than twice as likely to become demented as their vegetarian counterparts (Neuroepidemiology, 12:28-36, 1993)

Another recent study showed that subjects who adopted a vegan diet had their homocysteine levels drop between 13% and 20% in just ONE WEEK (Preventive Medicine 2000;30:225-233.)

OTHER DISEASES
A vegetarian diet has been claimed to also reduce the risk of gout, hiatus hernia, constipation, haemorrhoids, and varicose veins. These diseases are linked to diets low in fibre and high in saturated fat. Indeed, from if we start from the premise that flesh foods and animal products contain many and varied poisons and we realise that a build-up of poisons in our bodies result in ill-health, then we realise that flesh foods and animal products will always spell disease and ill-health and that a continuous build-up of poisons in the body will result, eventually, in serious ill-health.

CHAPTER SIXTEEN: DAIRY PRODUCTS

"Inclusion of milk will only reduce your diet's nutritional value and safety. Most of the people on the planet live very healthfully without cows milk. You can too." Robert M.Kradjian M.D

"I no longer recommend dairy products...there was a time when cow's milk was considered very desirable. But research along with clinical experience has forced doctors and nutritionists to rethink this recommendation"
Dr. Benjamin Spock

"Dairy foods are the most harmful of the traditional four food groups."
Dr. John McDougall

"I sometimes challenge milk drinkers by asking them if they would like a glass of milk containing 1,000 PUS CELLS. The average 12 ounce glass of milk in America contains 112,899,408 PUS CELLS." Robert Cohen - author of
Milk: The Deadly Poison

"There's no reason to drink cows milk at any time in your life. It was designed for calves, not humans and we should all stop drinking it today"
Dr. Frank A. Oski, former Director of Paediatrics, John Hopkins University

Since the main focus of this book discusses the relationship between flesh foods and disease, I will not go into too much detail as regards dairy products. However, it is doubtless that dairy products and other animal products also create major health problems amongst the human populations who consume them.

The evidence against cow's milk and the reports showing the relationship between cow's milk and a whole range of diseases and disorders are ever-increasing. According to Dr Colin Campbell(7) "There is compelling evidence, now published in top scientific journals and some of which is decades old, showing that cows' milk is associated, possibly even causally, with a wide variety of serious human ailments including various cancers, cardiovascular diseases, diabetes and an array of allergy-related diseases. And, this food contains no nutrients that cannot be better obtained from other far more nutritious and tasty foods.

A Good Source of Calcium?

Many people think that cow's milk builds strong bones and teeth, and that it is essential for good health due to the calcium content, however, this is not the case. Pasteurised animal milks are not fit food for humans. The only type of milk which is fit food for humans is the milk of our own species. Cow's milk is designed to build a small calf into a cow which is often why children on cow's milk grow to big so quickly. Cow's milk is for calves, and goat's milk is for kids - not human kids but kids of the goat variety! After children are weaned, at about three years of age in some, they no longer secrete the enzymes necessary to break down the casein (protein) or lactose (sugar) components of milk. This means that if we continue to consume milk, particularly milk from another species, it may lead to an array of disorders and intolerances and may cause some very severe health problems.

There are many sources of calcium which are far more beneficial than that of animal milk, without all the dangers to human health. In fact, **cow's milk causes more mucus than any food you can eat.** The casein in cow's milk can clog and irritates the body's entire respiratory system. Hay fever, asthma, bronchitis, sinusitis, colds, runny noses and ear infections are all caused by a consumption of dairy products. Dairy products are also the leading cause of allergies[1]. Casein, the protein component in milk, is a very thick and coarse substance and **is used to make one of the strongest glues known.** There is 300% more casein in cow's milk than there is in human's milk. By the age of three or four, the enzyme rennin needed to break down casein, is non-existent in the human body. **Dairy products are implicated in all respiratory problems.**

From their extensive research, Harvey and Marilyn Diamond conclude that dairy products aggravate ulcers, contribute to colitis, colon and prostate cancer, sudden infant death syndrome (SIDS), etc. They argue that the list of ailments that can be linked to dairy products is so extensive there is hardly a problem it doesn't at least contribute to [1].

154

One book that presents a most convincing and thorough indictment of dairy products is 'Don't Drink the Milk' by Oski and Bell. Included in the host of diseases and maladies which the authors attribute at least in part to dairy products are Lou Gehrig's disease and multiple sclerosis. Multiple sclerosis is most frequently found in areas of the world where children are raised on dairy products, rather than breast milk. A low animal fat diet used for thirty years by a medical doctor at the University of Oregon has dramatically helped multiple sclerosis patients.

Professor E. V. McCollum stressed the fact that cow's milk is <u>not</u> an essential in the diet of man. He pointed out that the inhabitants of Southern Asia never drink milk and that they have exceptionally well-developed physiques, and exceptional endurance and work capacity. They escape skeletal defects in childhood and have the finest teeth of any people in the world. Their diet is made up of rice, soya beans, sweet potatoes, bamboo sprouts and other vegetables. This is a sharp and favourable contrast with milk-drinking peoples([1]).

Industry Propoganda

Of course, due to propaganda fuelled by commercial interests, we consume far more protein than our bodies require. The RDA (Recommended Daily Allowance) is set at fifty-five grams per day, however, it has been shown that we only need about thirty grams a day. The World Health Organisation nearly double that figure to add a 'margin of safety' (on average, most people in the West are taking in about one hundred grams a day). We are led to believe that animal products are the best source of protein when it has been demonstrated over and over again that a diet totally devoid of animal products can supply us with all we need (Ibid.).

In 1930, the first study was published that showed that in humans a diet with a high meat content caused the loss of large amounts of calcium and a negative calcium balance. Eskimos consume one of the highest protein diets in the world, and they also have one of the highest incidences of osteoporosis in the world. They are already stooped over in their mid-twenties. The incidence of osteoporosis is lowest in the countries where the least amount of dairy products are consumed, and where protein consumption is highest, osteoporosis is most common (Ibid.). It has been shown clearly that when calcium is lost from the bones, which is often caused by excess protein in the diet, it is not just eliminated from the body. This calcium in the body is picked up by the blood and deposited in the soft tissues - the blood vessels, skin, eyes, joints and internal organs. As previously mentioned, excess (inorganic) calcium combines with fats and cholesterol in the blood vessels to cause hardening of the arteries, the excess which ends up in the skin causes wrinkles; in the joints calcium crystallises and forms very painful arthritic deposits; in the eyes it takes the form of cataracts and in the kidneys it forms hard deposits known as kidney stones (Ibid.).

The calcium-depleting effects of proteins are not lessened, even when large doses of calcium are ingested. What must be remembered is that calcium is found in all foods grown in the ground and that they supply a sufficient amount of calcium to meet the requirements of both growing children and adults. Animals consume the plants and absorb the calcium - THAT'S WHERE THE COW GETS CALCIUM!

Whilst there is iron in milk, only five-ten percent of it is available to the body and infants fed on cow's milk can suffer iron deficiency anaemia (Paediatrics, Volume 75, 1985, pp182). Other factors that contribute to a calcium intolerance are that milk is high in phosphorous (so is meat). Dairy milk has a harmful calcium/magnesium balance and high intakes of calcium depress calcitrol formation (a hormone produced in the body as a result of vitamin D absorption).

Conversely, the massive amount of dairy products that pregnant women are routinely terrorised into consuming is the reason why huge amounts of excess mucus coat infant's lungs and prevent them from developing properly. **Ever wondered why it's necessary to have a suction tube at every birth to suck the thick mucus from the infant's throat and nose immediately upon delivery so it can breath?** The January 1960 issue of The Lancet identifies the substance "muco-protein" in the lungs of infants who die of respiratory disease syndrome. This protein is precisely what develops in the body when dairy products are consumed and this substance coats the lungs of infants. It therefore follows that the respiratory disorders in young children and babies are often caused by dairy products.

The Physician's Committee for Responsible Medicine([2]) argue that dairy products are not required in the human diet. The main caloric constituents of dairy products are animal fat, animal protein, and lactose, none of which are required in the human diet. In fact, they argue that lactose maldigestion is biologically normal for adults of all mammalian species, and is common in most human populations. The potential health risks of the products of lactose digestion, particularly the role of lactose in the aetiology of cataracts and ovarian problems, are an area of ongoing research.

Those who advocate milk consumption do so, not on the basis of its supposed macronutrients, but because of its supposed micronutrients: calcium and supplemental vitamin D. However, other more healthful sources of calcium and vitamin D are available. More importantly, calcium balance involves far more than calcium intake. Dietary changes that reduce calcium losses are probably much more important for us.

Cancer
Recent research into cancer of the ovaries has established a connection between animal fat and cancer. The PCRM say that there was a significant trend towards the increasing risk of ovarian cancer with increasing animal fat consumption and one study found that women who consume the most animal fat in their diet run *double* the risk of contracting ovarian cancer when compared to those who consume the least (Ibid.). In a recent article published by the PCRM([3]). Saroja Koneswaran M.D. and Gowri Koneswaran argue that dairy products have been linked to breast cancer. Apparently, the hormone oestrogen increases the risk and milk is filled with the oestrogen of the mother cow who produced it.

Diabetes and Multiple Sclerosis
More recently, studies have shown links between drinking cow's milk and both juvenile diabetes and multiple sclerosis in Canada([5]). In an

article entitled 'Researchers Link Cows' Milk to Juvenile Diabetes and MS' it was reported that drinking cows' milk may be a risk factor for multiple sclerosis as well as juvenile diabetes, two diseases Canadian researchers have discovered as being remarkably similar. Dr. Michael Dosch, Senior Scientist at the Hospital for Sick Children in Toronto said he and other researchers suspect that infants who are genetically predisposed to diabetes are at greater risk of getting the disease if they are given formula - which is usually based on cows' milk - before they are three months old. The researchers don't know at what age drinking cows' milk may have an impact on multiple sclerosis, however, they do know that both MS patients and diabetics in recent tests shared an abnormal immune-system response to cows' milk.

Multiple sclerosis is a disease of the central nervous system - the brain and spinal cord - which can leave patients using a wheelchair. Diabetes affects the pancreas. Patients are unable to regulate blood levels of glucose, a sugar our cells need for energy. Without insulin, diabetics can lapse into a coma or die. Both are termed medically as 'autoimmune diseases', which means they happen because the body's immune system attacks its own tissue, and both have a genetic component as well as environmental risk factors. In MS, the immune system destroys the protective lining around nerve cells. The idea would be to prevent damage before it becomes too serious. The researchers discovered that in both diseases, T-cells, the big guns of our immune system, run amok attacking healthy tissue. Not only that, but in the laboratory, the T-cells from diabetics will attack central nervous system proteins, and the T-cells from MS patients will go after pancreatic proteins. 'We found that both tissues are targetted in each disease', Dr. Dosch said.

Osteoporosis
The PCRM say that 40 million American women suffer from the effects of bone disease. They refer to a Harvard study([6]) of 78,000 nurses, who drank three or more glasses of milk per day and still did not reduce fractures at all. An Australian study showed the same thing. The Journal of Epidemiology published a case-controlled study of risk factors for hip fractures in the elderly. This study concludes: "Consumption of dairy products, particularly at age 20 years, were

158

associated with an increased risk of hip fractures." The Australian study provides the mechanism for such a high correlation. The authors explain that the metabolism of dietary protein causes increased urinary excretion of calcium.

And a Host of Other Diseases!

Dr Julian Whitaker[8] argues that cow's milk is species-specific food for calves. It is no more appropriate to drink the milk of cows than it is to drink the milk of other mammals. He argues that there are many myths surrounding milk-drinking and that misguided nutritionists reinforce it. Apart from the osteoporotic state that milk induces, as mentioned, he argues that dairy products are clearly linked as a cause of heart disease, obesity, cancer, allergies and diabetes and that dairy products are anything but "health" foods. The association with heart disease is particularly strong. He also cites a study by Dr Grant which summarises the mounting evidence that non-fat milk is also a major player in bringing on heart disease. Writing in Alternative Medicine Review, Dr. Grant points out that non-fat milk, which contains substantial amounts of dairy protein, is also very low in B vitamins. The metabolism of all the protein in milk and the absence of B vitamins contributes to the build-up of homocysteine, a marker for heart disease.

Dr Whitaker further argues that there are three reasons kids and milk don't mix. First, milk is the leading cause of iron-deficiency anaemia in infants, and, in fact, the American Academy of Pediatrics now discourages giving children milk before their first birthday. Second, it has been shown that milk consumption in childhood contributes to the development of Type-I diabetes. Certain proteins in milk resemble molecules on the beta cells of the pancreas that secrete insulin. In some cases, the immune system makes antibodies to the milk protein that mistakenly attack and destroy the beta cells.

Dr Whitaker argues that milk allergies are very common in children and cause sinus problems, diarrhoea, constipation and fatigue. They are a leading cause of the chronic ear infections that plague up to 40% of all children under the age of six. Milk allergies are also linked to behaviour problems in children and to the disturbing rise of childhood asthma. (Milk allergies are equally common in adults and produce similar symptoms.)

"In only two generations, the rate of hip fractures in the U.S. has quadrupled, and it is currently one of the highest rates in the world. Americans are also near the top of the chart for dairy consumption. Would someone out there please tell me why we keep telling our children that dairy foods strengthen their bones? Excess protein intake - not only from milk but all animal protein sources increases the need for calcium to neutralise acidic protein breakdown products, destroying bone in the process. A lifetime of a high-protein diet usually eats away at your bones. Lower protein vegetarian diets are associated with significantly higher bone mineral density. So the first and most important dietary step is to eat less protein. This generally means cutting down on milk..." Dr Julian Whitaker

Of course, we do need a supply of calcium in our diet, and good non-dairy sources include green leafy vegetables, raw nuts and seeds and carrots. In fact all vegetables contain calcium and so do many fruits. The amount of calcium you need from your diet will decrease when you eliminate salt and animal protein from your diet. Regular exercise and adequate vitamin D (from day light and sunshine) are also important factors too.

CHAPTER SEVENTEEN: EGGS

EXPLODING THE MYTHS!

The adverts are everywhere - eggs are a good source of nutrients, but is this true? Let's examine some of the most recent scientific evidence.

If we think about, most commercial hens which are bred for egg production are hardly healthy animals. They are fed antibiotics, hormones, yolk colourants, artificial additives and other questionable substances such as arsenic(!) to kill parasites and stimulate egg production as well as the fact that their food is laced with pesticides. Salmonella is highly prevalent in commercial flocks of hens, as is campylobacter and contaminated eggs have been proven to cause food poisoning in people. In fact, in a study carried out in the U.S. in 1985-88, eggs were responsible for salmonella outbreaks affecting 5,000 people, 898 of whom had to be hospitalised as a result.

Egg yolks contain a whopping 213 mg of cholesterol each, which constitutes more than 70% of the maximum recommended daily intake and serving up just one egg for breakfast each morning can raise your cholesterol level by as much as 10 points! We synthesise about 1500mg of cholesterol per day within our bodies and simply do not need any extra cholesterol in our diet. This is why it's hardly surprising that many experts speak out against egg consumption and it's consumption to heart disease. It has also recently been discovered that women who eat eggs daily triple their risk of breast cancer.

In a recent article by 'The American Journal of Clinical Nutrition' in a study entitled: 'Eating Fewer Eggs Still Good for Heart' states that although in recent years conflicting studies on the effects of eggs on health have sent consumers scrambling for some definitive answers, a new study reports that even though eggs can boost HDL ("good") cholesterol, they also raise total cholesterol even more. The bottom line, write researchers in the May 2000 issue of the 'American Journal of Clinical Nutrition', is that people should limit egg consumption to reduce their risk of heart disease. `The advice to limit cholesterol intake by reducing consumption of eggs and other cholesterol-rich foods may...still be valid," concludes lead author Rianne M. Weggemans and colleagues from Wageningen University in the Netherlands. Their review of 17 medical studies involving 556 individuals found that adding 100 milligrams (mg) of cholesterol to the diet each day, the equivalent of half an egg, increased the ratio of total cholesterol to HDL cholesterol in the blood. The investigators used this ratio to account for any beneficial effect that was found for HDL cholesterol.

Cholesterol, found in animal foods such as meat and dairy products has, in some studies, been shown to increase both total cholesterol and LDL ("bad") cholesterol, which contribute to heart disease risk. The overall evidence seems to weigh in against unlimited egg consumption, the researchers conclude. ``In view of the relatively small contribution of eggs to the intake of these nutrients, the recommendation to limit the consumption of eggs may still be valid for the prevention of coronary heart disease," Weggemans and colleagues write.

Furthermore, laboratory tests carried out by the Eclipse Scientific Group I in Cambridge, England on free-range eggs show that even with so-called free-range hens, chemicals are being fed to hens to make their egg yolks appear a deeper yellow. Two of the colourants citranaxanthin (E161i) and Beta-Apo 8 Carotenal (E160), are approved by the egg industries lion code, but Canthaxanthin (E161g) found in eggs imported from Germany by the Lidl discount chain, has been linked to eye defects. Although this chemical is banned from human foods, it is still legal to use it in hen feed (Daily Mail, 20.11.99).

You may be wondering if eggs fare any better than flesh foods as a source for protein. However, high-quality protein is not what we should search for; high-quality amino acids are what we need to produce the protein we must have. Unless eggs are eaten raw, the amino acids are coagulated by eat and thereby lost, but obviously raw eggs are more likely to contain the potentially deadly salmonella bug.

Another side to the egg debate is that eggs are unnaturally high in sulphur. According to Dr Robert Young, a microbiologist and nutritionist from the U.S., in his book 'Sick and Tired', sulphuric acid is capable of burning a whole through your clothing so it requires special handling and you will find sulphuric acid in eggs and in your car's battery. You know you wouldn't drink battery acid, so why would you eat an egg, he asks? Added to this, Dr Young reports that 15 minutes after eating an egg, our bloodstream will show the presence or high increase of bacteria. Eggs from grain-fed chickens has been found to contain more mycotoxins[2].

According to Harvey and Marilyn Diamond, eggs are neither a valuable food nor are they a health food. Remember what all health professionals are recommending that we do? Less fat and cholesterol and more fibre. Eggs are very high in fat and cholesterol and contain essentially no fibre. **In fact, ounce for ounce, eggs contain 8 times more cholesterol than beef!** The egg industry denies all of the negatives about eggs in much the same way that the Tobacco Industry defends itself. Dr John McDougall points to only 6 studies in medical literature that show that eggs don't dramatically affect blood cholesterol levels, three of which were funded by the American Egg Board, one by the Missouri Egg Merchandising Council, one by the Egg Programme of the California Department of Agriculture (the sixth is not identified). As Dr McDougall states, "The Egg Industry provides a timely example of how money can buy scientific nutritional information that can be detrimental to your health"[3].

So if you're still eating eggs and you're worried about your health, why not try replacing eggs with plant foods which are rich in protein (amino acids) such as nuts, seeds, legumes (sprouted preferably), beans or pulses, not forgetting green leafy vegetables?

CONCLUSION:
HEALTH AND A PLANT- BASED DIET

The reader has now seen that a plant-based diet is known to confer a wide range of health benefits. Research has shown vegetarians to suffer less heart disease, hypertension, obesity, diabetes, various cancers, diverticular disease, bowel disorders, gallstones, kidney stones, and osteoporosis. Vegetarian diets have also been used in the treatment of various illnesses, including rheumatoid arthritis and nephrotic syndrome. Dickerson and Davies[1] studied matched pairs of vegetarians and non-vegetarians with regard to their general health. It was found that the vegetarians made 22% of the visits to hospital out-patients, as compared to non-vegetarians, and spent a similarly reduced proportion of time in hospital.

Yet for many years we have been told that we must have lots of protein and calcium in our diet and, we are told, meat and animal products are our way of providing this. In reality, meat (including fish and fowl) is the hardest thing for the human body to digest, as the reader would have noted. Consumption of such foods result in poor health, sooner or later. This is because the human body is not designed anatomically, physiologically or bio-chemically to consume flesh foods or flesh products. Cooked animal protein causes a great drain on our energy supplies and leaves us feeling fatigued and helps us on our way to degenerative disease.

The consumption of this type of food results in an inevitable putrefaction and the resultant poisonous by-products play havoc with our health. The human body can take in sufficient nutrients when the food we eat is whole, raw and plant. I repeat, a diet consisting of mainly or solely raw plant foods should give us ALL THE NUTRIENTS WE NEED (providing we do not have a malabsorption syndrome) and is all the body requires for its vital functioning.

Of course, a typical plant-based diet closely matches expert dietary recommendations for healthy eating, being low in saturated fat and high in fibre and fresh fruit and vegetables. The 1983 NACNE Report

(National Advisory Committee on Nutrition Education) in the UK recommended a reduction in fat intake, particularly saturated fat, and an increased dietary proportion of polyunsaturated fats to saturated fats. An increased intake of complex carbohydrates and fibre and a decreased intake of sugar and salt were also recommended.

The World Health Organisation (1990) has similarly recommended a reduced intake of fat and increased consumption of complex carbohydrates. Increased consumption of fruit, vegetables, cereals and pulses is also recommended. The nutritional guidelines from the World Health Organisation, the NACNE Report and other expert bodies form the basis of advice given on healthy eating by leading health professionals today. Vegetarian diets tend to be lower in total fat. (Millet, 1989).

Vegetarians also tend to eat proportionally more polyunsaturated fat to saturated fat compared with non-vegetarians. Animal products are the major sources of dietary saturated fat. Also, recent research has demonstrated the importance of protective antioxidant nutrients in the diet, found in fresh fruits and vegetables. These antioxidant nutrients include the beta-carotene form of vitamin A, vitamin C and E. Many researchers now believe that these nutrients play a major role in reducing the risk of chronic diseases such as heart disease and cancer. A high consumption of fresh fruit and vegetables is the tremendous benefit of a plant-based diet.

So there we have it, study after study conclusively proving that a low-fat, plant-based diet, rich in fresh fruits and vegetables is a major factor in the prevention of many and varied diseases. This book has shown time and time again studies revealing that fact that meat is poisonous to the human body and that a strict vegetarian diet, to which we are adapted to, can not only prevent but also reverse acute and degenerative disease.

The China Project on Nutrition, Health and Environment is a massive study involving researchers from China, Cornell University in Boston, and the University of Oxford, into the relationships between diet, lifestyles and disease-related mortality in 6,500 Chinese subjects from sixty-five mostly rural or semi-rural counties([1]). The rural Chinese diet is largely vegetarian or vegan, and involves less total protein, less animal protein, less total fat and animal fat, and more carbohydrate and fibre than the average Western diet. Blood cholesterol levels are significantly lower. Heart disease, cancer, obesity, diabetes, and osteoporosis are all uncommon. Areas in which they are becoming more frequent are areas where the population has moved towards a more Western diet, with increasing consumption of animal products. The China Health Project has clearly demonstrated the health benefits of a diet based on plant foods. One of the Project's co-ordinators, Dr Colin Campbell of Cornell University, has stated that "We're basically a vegetarian species and should be eating a wide variety of plant foods and minimising our intake of animal foods."

When we adopt a vegan diet, naturally, health in general will improve even more. In the instance of those people who subsist on a mainly raw food diet, health will improve dramatically. The reason for this is simple. Our bodies are not designed to eat cooked food and it is at great expense to the body that we subsist on cooked foods. Vitality dwindles, energy levels decrease and sleep needs rise dramatically when we try to survive on a cooked food diet. This food either has to be eliminated as quickly as possible, having taken whatever nutrients it can find from it, or else stored in adipose tissue.

However, upon switching to a raw food and juices diet many people have allowed their bodies to heal from life-threatening diseases such as various forms of cancer, heart disease, diabetes, arthritis, chronic fatigue syndrome, etc. Many have also turned around the ageing process.

Scientific evidence shows that raw vegan diets decrease toxic products in the colon (J Nutr 1992 Apr;122(4):924-30). Shifting from a conventional diet to an uncooked vegan diet reversibly alters faecal hydrolytic activities in humans, according to researchers, Ling WH, and Hanninen O, of the Department of Physiology, University of Kuopio, Finland. Results suggest a raw food uncooked vegan diet causes a decrease in bacterial enzymes and certain toxic products that have been implicated in colon cancer risk. Researchers that a diet rich in raw vegetables also lowers your risk of breast cancer, and that eating lots of fruit reduces your risk for colon cancer, according to a study published in the May 1998 issue of the journal Epidemiology. Including fresh fruit as part of your daily diet has been associated with fewer deaths from heart attacks and related problems, by as much as 24%, according to a study published in the September 1996 issue of the British Medical Journal.

As previously mentioned research shows that adding fire to food causes dangerous changes in the food structure, including the creation of carcinogenic substances. According to research performed by cancerologist Dr. Bruce Ames, professor of Biochemistry and Molecular Biology at University of California, Berkeley various groups of chemicals from cooked food causes tumors: Nitrosamines are created from fish, poultry or meat cooked in gas ovens and barbecues, as nitrogen oxides within gas flames interact with fat residues· Hetrocyclic amines form from heating proteins and amino acids; Polycyclic hydrocarbons are created by charring meat; Mucoid plaque, a thick tar-like substance builds up in the intestines on a diet of cooked foods. Mucoid plaque is caused by uneliminated, partically digested, putrefying cooked fatty and starch foods eaten in association with protein flesh foods; Lipofuscin is another toxin: an accumulation of waste materials throughout the body and within cells of the skin, manifesting as age-spots; in the liver as liver-spots; and in the nervous system including the brain, possibly contributing to ossification of gray matter and senility.

From the book Diet, Nutrition and Cancer published by the Nutritional Research Council of the American Academy of Sciences (1982) and the FDA (Food and Drug Administration) Office of Toxicological Sciences, additional carcinogens in heated foods include: Hydroperoxide, alkoxy, endoperoxides and epoxides from heated meat, eggs, fish and pasteurized milk; Ally aldehyde (acrolein), butyric acid, nitropyrene, nitrobenzene and nitrosamines from heated fats and oils; Methyglyoxal and chlorogenic atractyosides in coffee; Indole, skatole, nitropyrene, ptomatropine, ptomaines, leukomaines, ammonia, hydrogen sulfide, cadaverine, muscarine, putecine, nervine, and mercaptins in cheese.

According to Arthur Baker, a health educator from the U.S., three important changes immediately occur when you adopt a raw food diet. First is the improved quality of nutrients taken into your system. Raw fresh produce is nutrient dense, largely pre-digested nutriment that is easily absorbed into your blood. Heated nutrients are denatured and of inferior quality, which are among the reasons why people commonly overeat cooked food. While their stomach feels full, their physiology craves nutrients and remains nutritionally starved.

The second important change that occurs on raw food cuisine involves what you STOP eating. No longer introduced into your system are devitalized, refined, heat-damaged toxic nutrient remnants. Energy is no longer wasted that previously was devoted to flushing these nutrient antagonists away from cells and tissues or quarantining them into fat cells, cysts, warts or tumors and abnormal growths. Instead, this energy is now redirected to enhance internal cleansing and further maximize the unfoldment of wellness.

The third major change on a fresh produce diet is the cessation of overeating. Overeating saturates the body with degenerated unnatural foodstuffs that constipate or clog the bloodstreams nutrient delivery and sewage cleansing system. The blood delivers nutrients and oxygen to living cells, and carries away their toxic metabolites generated during ordinary cellular metabolism. This is why obesity is a serious condition. With too much food, the body is overburdened with inferior nutritionless empty calories.

High fibre, high water content fresh produce abolishes constipation of the bowels, cells and circulatory system. Obstructions are cleared and blood flow increases to each and every cell in the body. Enhanced blood flow is significant for two reasons: as mentioned above, blood delivers nutrients and oxygen to living cells, and carries away their toxic metabolites(4).

Raw food, as mentioned throughout this book, is the optimum diet for humankind. Fired foods lose their nutrient content by up to eighty percent and their protein usability by approximately fifty percent.

Cooking also destroys 60-70% of the vitamins, up to 96% of the B12, and 100% of many of the lesser factors like gibberellins, anthrocyans, nobelitin, and tangeretin which boost the immune system and other body functions. Another very important factor behind a high raw diet is that of enzymes. Cooking of foods destroys their enzyme content which means that the body has to use up its own supply of enzymes, which uses up our vital energy. According to Dr Paul Kouchakoff, every time we eat cooked food, our bodies produce a proliferation of white blood cells to get rid of the invader![2] This does not happen when we eat raw plant foods.

Indeed, further studies have emerged this year where scientists have reported again that heating foods such as starches, sugars and fats produce possible carcinogens compounds. The article, entitled 'Cancer Chemicals in Most Cooked Foods'[3], reported that a chemical suspected of causing cancer has been found in most of the cooked food we eat. It states that British scientists report that significant levels of acrylamide occur in a wide range of processed and cooked foods. Their study focussed on chips, crisps, breakfast cereals and rye crispbreads but experts say that other food such as meat may be at risk. The article goes on to say that acrylamide forms naturally in food when it is fried or baked. Frying for longer than usual increased levels of the chemical. Researchers believe it is also found in roasted, grilled and barbecued food.

Anatomically and physiologically, as detailed herein, human beings are frugivores and can only live healthfully on a diet primarily consisting of fresh, ripe raw fruit, nuts and seeds and green leafy vegetables. Raw plant material is the only thing our bodies' recognise as food and eating this way is the only way to achieve maximum vitality and optimum health.

So, in conclusion, we have found that a meat-based diet is not desirable for health and that the diet most suited to our biological adaptation is one of plant foods only, preferably in their whole, raw state.

Bibliography

SECTION ONE
INTRODUCTION
1. 'Toxic Meal Syndrome' by Patrice Green, J.D., M.D. and Allison Lee Solin of PCRM, August 2000
2. 'High Dioxin Levels Found in Food' ABC News , 30 March 2001
3. 'Risk of Death from Cancer and Ischaemic Heart Disease in Meat and non-Meat Eaters' BMJ, 1994, Issue 308
4. 'Meat Your Death?', Jacobs, L. J. (M.D.) and Kweller, C. - May 2001 - www.pcrm.org
5. 'Our Voice', 5th Ed., The Nutritional Cancer Therapy Trust, March 2001
6. 'Sick and Tired', Young, R and Redford Young, S., Woodland Publishing; January 2000
7. 'Hormone Deception', Lindsey Berkson, D., 2000 - Contemporary Books

CHAPTER ONE: SCIENTIFIC REASONS FOR AVOIDING MEAT
1. The Life Science Institute Course in Natural Health (Canada), 1986
2. What's Wrong with Eating Meat?, 1981 - Sisters Universal Publishing
3. The Price of Meat, Penman, D., 1996 - Victor Gollancz Publications
4. The Higher Taste, 1983 - The Bhaktivedanta Book Trust
5. Raw Energy, Kenton, L. and S., 1987 - Arrow Books
6. 'Controlling Cholesterol', Physicians Committee for Responsible Medicine Article, PCRM Website, August 2000
7. 'Hormone Deception', Lindsey Berkson, D., 2000 - Contemporary Books
8. 'Paleolithic Nutrition', Boyd ES and Konner M, 1985 - New Eng J Med, 312, 283-289
9. 'The Pritikin Promise', Pritikin, N, 1985 - Bantam Books

CHAPTER TWO: THE VITAMIN B12 ISSUE
1. The Life Science Institute Course in Natural Health (Canada), 1986
2. The Encyclopaedia of Vegetarian Living, Cox, P., 1994 - Bloomsbury Publications
3. 'Fit for Life', Diamond, H. and M., 1987
4. 'Nutrition and Athletic Performance', Graham, Dr. G., 1999
5. 'Female Balance' article on www.living-foods.com, Fierro, K., 2001
6. 'Human Anatomy and Physiology', Marieb, 1999
7. Correspondence with Dr Vetrano's family - 2001
8. 'The Sunfood Diet Success Story', Wolfe, D, 2000
9. Vitamin B12 internet article, The Vegan Society, 2001
10. Vitamin B12, internet article, The Vegetarian Society, 2001
11. Vitamin B12, 'Solstice Magazine' article, 1990
12. 'Female Balance' article on www.living-foods.com, Fierro, K., 2001
13. 'Human Anatomy and Physiology', Marieb, 1999
14 Correspondence with Dr Vetrano's family - 2001
15 'The Sunfood Diet Success Story', Wolfe, D, 2000

16 Vitamin B12 internet article, The Vegan Society, 2001
17 Vitamin B12, internet article, The Vegetarian Society, 2001
18 Vitamin B12, 'Solstice Magazine' article, 1990
19 'Vitamin B12', 'In Balance' Autumn 1999/Issue 30, Rofe, A. - Vegan Society
20 'Vitamin, Mineral and Dietary Supplements', Walji, 1998
21 'Vitamins for Dummies' - 1998
22 Marcus et al, J Am Geriatr Soc 35;635-8; 1987
23 Vitamin B12 in Present Knowledge in Nutrition', Herbert, V, 7th Ed., Elselvier Press, pp195-6
24 Raising Kids Vegan - Will it Lead to Learning Impairment?'', Root, M. (PhD) and Nelson, J., www.vegsource.com May 2001
25 'Female Balance' article on www.living-foods.com, Fierro, K., 2001
26 Pregnancy, Children and the Vegan Diet', Klaper (MD), M, Gentle World;(May 1988)
27 Conscious Eating', Cousens, Dr G., North Atlantic Books; January 15, 2000
28 Dietary Aspects of Vitamin B12', Berkowsky, B, British Naturopathic Journal – 1998
29 Sick and Tired', Young, R and Redford Young, Dr S., Woodland Publishing; January 2000
30 The Vegetarian Option: Heretical or Healthy?, Ryde, Dr D, The British Holistic Medical Association

CHAPTER THREE: THE PROTEIN MYTH

1. Raw Energy, Kenton, L. and S., 1987 - Arrow Books
1. The Life Science Institute Course in Natural Health (Canada), 1986
2. Radical Rejuvenation, Dillon, R., 1996 - Headline Book Publishing
3. Fit for Life Living Health, Diamond, H and M, 1992 - Bantam Books
5. Vegsource.com article April 2001
6. Gerson Healing Newsletter Vol. 16, No.2, Mar-April 2001

SECTION TWO
CHAPTER FOUR: THE DANGERS OF EATING SHEEP AND LAMBS

1. The Price of Meat, Penman, D.., 1996 - Victor Gollancz Publications
2. VIVA! Magazine, Winter 1999/2000
3. Its the Silence of the Lambs', Thursday, March 22, 2001, Alvarez, M. and Perrotta, K., New York Times Online

CHAPTER FIVE: THE DANGERS OF EATING PIG MEAT

1. The Price of Meat, Penman, D., 1996 - Victor Gollancz Publications
2. PCRM Article "Frankly, You Should Give a Damn" by Neal D. Barnard, M.D., and A.R. Hogan, August 2000
3. 'Don't Eat Any Babe' PCRM Health Commentary by Neal D. Barnard, M.D. and Karen Pirozzi, December 1998
4. 'AIDS-Like Symptoms Threaten Pigs', ABCNEWS.com, 29th March 2001

CHAPTER SIX: FISH AND SEAFOOD - THE _UNHEALTHY_ OPTION

1. "Fishy Business" Article by Sue Dibbs of The Food Commission, 1997
2. Pisces Information Sheet, 1997
3. Article by John Andrews, Health Action Network, 1997
4. "Its Purely Personal" Article by Joy Hetherington (The Vegetarian 1997)
5. The Society for the Promotion of Nutritional Therapy Newsletter, Spring 2000
6. Article by Neal Barnard (MD) in Animal Times, Summer 2000
7. "The One That Got Away: New Seafood Regulations Come up Short" by Neal D. Barnard, M.D., and Cindy S. Spitzer, July 1998
8. New York Times, April 2001
9. CNN Health Report entitled 'Fish-Mercury Risk Under-Estimated' April 12, 2001
10. KIRO-7 Eyewitness News Consumer Reporter - 5th June 2001
11. 'Hormone Deception', Lindsey Berkson, D., 2000 - Contemporary Books

CHAPTER SEVEN WHAT EVERYONE SHOULD KNOW ABOUT POULTRY MEAT

1. Farm Animal Welfare Network Fact Sheet 37 - January 1994
2. The Higher Taste, 1983 - The Bhaktivedanta Book Trust
3. "Eating Responsibly in the Age of the Epidemic' Article by Murry Cohen, M.D., and Allison Lee Solin of the PCRM (in 'Commentary of the Month"), August 2000
4. Physicians Committee for Responsible Medicine "Commentary of the Month" Have (Healthy) Heart; Go Vegetarian' by Neal D. Barnard, M.D., and A.R.Hogan, March 1999
5. There's No Room for Chicken in a Healthy Diet' by Kristine Kieswer, PCRM Magazine, Spring/Summer 2000 (Volume IX, Number 2)"
6. 'Chicken: Run Away' by Dr Barnard and K Keiswer (PCRM Health Commentary), September 2000
7. 'Chicken the Healthy Option' leaflet, 1999, by VIVA!, Brighton, England
8. 'Intensive Egg, Chicken and Turkey Production' - (Undated Publication) - Chicken's Lib, c/o Animal Aid, Tonbridge, Kent.
9. 'UK Watchdog Says Shop Chickens Rife with Food Bug' 16th August 2001, www.dailynews.yahoo.com - August 2001
10. 'Hormone Deception', Lindsey Berkson, D., 2000 - Contemporary Books

CHAPTER EIGHT: CAN ANIMAL DISEASES SPREAD TO HUMANS?

1. The Encyclopaedia of Vegetarian Living, Cox, P.,1994 - Bloomsbury Publication
2. The New Why You Don't Need Meat, Cox, P, 1994-Bloomsbury Publications
3. Why You Don't Need Meat, Cox, P., 1992 - Bloomsbury Publishing

CHAPTER NINE: HEALTH RISKS RELATED TO BEEF AND VEAL

1. 'The Price of Meat', Penman, D.,1996 - Victor Gollancz Publications
2. 'CJD Claims 100th Victim' - BBC News - 24th May 2001
3. 'You Don't Have to Feel Unwell!', Bottomley, R - Newleaf Publishing – 1994

SECTION THREE
CHAPTER TEN: ARTHRITIS AND RHEUMATISM
1. The Encyclopaedia of Vegetarian Living, Cox, P., 1994 - Bloomsbury Publications
2. The Life Science Institute Course in Natural Health (Canada), 1986

CHAPTER ELEVEN: OSTEOPOROSIS
1. The Encyclopaedia of Vegetarian Living, Cox, P., 1994 - Bloomsbury Publications
2. PCRM - September 1995 News Release
3. Fit for Life Living Health, Diamond, H and M., 1992 - Bantam Books
4. The Life Science Institute Course in Natural Health (Canada), 1986
5. What the Doctors Don't Tell You, McTaggart, L., 1996 - Thorsons

CHAPTER TWELVE: MEAT, LEUKAEMIA AND CANCER
1. Fit for Life Living Health, Diamond, H. and M., 1992 - Bantam Books
2. The Encyclopaedia of Vegetarian Living, Cox, P, 1994 - Bloomsbury Publications
3. PCRM Article, 'The Vegan', Summer 1997
4. PCRM, September 1995 News Release
5. PCRM Article "Getting a Head Start in the Race against Prostate Cancer" by Neal D. Barnard, M.D., and A.R. Hogan, February 1999
6. 'Diet and Prostate Cancer' Article, PCRM Website Dr J. Whitaker Website (www.julian-whitaker.com) - 2000
7. Raw Energy, Kenton, L. and S., 1987 - Arrow Books
8. The Life Science Institute Course in Natural Health (Canada) – 1986
9. 'Diet, Nutrition and Cancer', 1982 - the Nutritional Research Council of the American Academy of Sciences

CHAPTER THIRTEEN: DIABETES
1. The Encyclopaedia of Vegetarian Living, Cox, P, 1994 - Bloomsbury Publications
2. PCRM September 1995 News Release
3. Radical Rejuvenation, Dillon, R., 1996 - Headline Book Publishing
4. Raw Energy, Kenton, L. and S., 1987 - Arrow Books
5. 'Can a Vegan Diet Cure Diabetes?' article by Andrew Nicholson, M.D., The Vegan, Summer 1997

CHAPTER FOURTEEN: HEART DISEASE AND HYPERTENSION
1. PCRM September 1995 News Release
2. The Encyclopaedia of Vegetarian Living, Cox, .,1994-Bloomsbury Publishing
3. Fit for Life Living Health, Diamond, H. and M., 1992 - Bantam Books
4. The Life Science Institute Course in Natural Health (Canada), 1986
5. 'Have a (Healthy) Heart; Go Vegetarian' article by Neal D. Barnard, MD. and A.R. Hogan, March 1999
6. 'Hypertension: The Answers on the Tip of your Tongue' Article by PCRM, October 1998

7. 'Eat Like The Apes', Beck, L, Toronto Star, Canada - 2001

CHAPTER FIFTEEN: OTHER HUMAN CONDITIONS & HEALTH PROBLEMS & THEIR RELATIONSHIP TO MEAT-CONSUMPTION
1. PCRM September 1995 News Release
2. PCRM Article 'Nutritional Factors in Menstrual Pain and Premenstrual Syndrome' by Neal D. Barnard, M.D. , 2000
3. 'Treating Multiple Sclerosis with Diet: Fact or Fraud?' by John A. McDougall, M.D. from PCRM Website reprinted from Vegetarian Times, Oak Park, Illinois, USA
4. 'Losing Your Mind for the Sake of a Burger', Nelson, J., www.vegsource.com February 2001
5. News item from www.alzheimer2000.org/news - early 2001

CHAPTER SIXTEEN: DAIRY PRODUCTS
1. Fit for Life Living Health - Diamond, H. and M., 1992 - Bantam Books
2. PCRM September 1995 News Release
3. 'U.S. Dietary Guidelines: A Recipe for Disease in the Melting Pot' Article by Koneswaran, Dr S., and Koneswaran, G , PCRM Health Commentary, October 1999
4. 'Milk: The Deadly Poison', Cohen, R. - Argus Publishing, Inc., Englewood Cliffs, NJ, 1998)
5. 'Researchers Link Cows' Milk To Juvenile Diabetes and MS', McIlroy, A - The Globe and Mail, Canada - March 21, 2001 (source www.Vegsource.com)
6. From www.notmilk.com April 2001 Newsletter, quoting PCRM's reference to 'The Harvard Nurse's study' - Cumming & Klineberg, published in the American Journal of Epidemiology & the Australian study - Feskanich, published in the American Journal of Public Health.
7. New Century Nutrition article, Campbell, Dr. C., www.vegsource.com - April 2001
8. 'What Dr Whitaker says about Dairy', www.notmilk.com - Dairy Education Board - May 2001

CHAPTER SEVENTEEN: EGGS
1. 'Eating Fewer Eggs Still Good for Heart', The American Journal of Clinical Nutrition' May 2001;73:885-891
2. 'Sick and Tired', Young, Dr R and Redford Young, S., Woodland Publishing; January 2000
3. Fit for Life Living Health, Diamond, H and M, 1992 - Bantam Books

CONCLUSION: HEALTH AND A PLANT-BASED DIET
1. Vegetarian Society "Health and Vegetarians" Pamphlet – 1999
2. Raw Energy, Kenton, L. and S., 1987 - Arrow Books
3. 'Cancer Chemicals in Most Cooked Foods' 18th May 2002, Daily Mirror
4. 'Raw Fresh Produce vs. Cooked Are Humans an Exception?' Baker, Art - 2001 www.healthcreation.net